D1016963

FIRM for LIFE

FIRM for LIFE

A Lifelong Plan for Fitness, Energy, and Overall Good Health

From the creators of
America's #1 fitness videos, The **FIRM**®

Anna and Cynthia Benson

BROADWAY BOOKS   NEW YORK

BROADWAY

Broadway Books titles may be purchased for business or promotional use or for
special sales. For information, please write to: Special Markets Department, Bantam
Doubleday Dell Publishing Group, Inc., 1540 Broadway, New York, NY 10036.

BROADWAY BOOKS and its logo, a letter B bisected on the diagonal, are trademarks
of Broadway Books, a division of Bantam Doubleday Dell Publishing Group, Inc.

ISBN 0-7679-0174-6

The FIRM and FIRM Believers are registered trademarks.

Designed by Michael Mendelsohn of MM Design 2000, Inc.

To those who helped make this possible:

Our partner and Anna's husband, Mark Henriksen, who ensured our video productions were award-winning and without whom our ventures would have been impossible;

Our parents for giving us so many enriching opportunities to learn and for teaching us that fulfilling work is a true blessing;

The original FIRM Believers whom we've never met but who financed The FIRM video library when bankers wouldn't;

The new FIRM Believers, who continue to make all our efforts worthwhile;

The South Carolina FIRM instructors and clients, who set daily examples of true beauty and leadership;

And, from Cynthia, to her husband, Sam, for his understanding and patience with my work, and for inspiring me daily with his generosity of spirit and loving kindnesses.

CONTENTS

CONTENTS

ACKNOWLEDGMENTS

We would like to thank the following for their contributions to this book: at our office to Janet Brunson, Tara Judge, Cathy Sovde, Mark Ross, Betty Coker, and Bernie Bernhagen for coordination and support into the late hours; at Broadway Books to Lauren Marino for her vision and to Kati Steele for her dedicated support; at Callwood-Tahir and Associates to Ahmed Tahir for his insightful representation; to Carolyn Fireside, whose work was invaluable; at BMG Video, to the fine folks who have been so generous and supportive of this project.

CHAPTER 1

FIRM
foundations

Hello—we're Anna and Cynthia Benson, creators of The FIRM, America's #1 exercise videos. Nine of the top ten bestselling health and fitness videos listed in recent issues of *Billboard Magazine* were designed by The FIRM. The FIRM has repeatedly received top scores in video ratings by over twenty national publications, including *Self, Shape,* and *American Health.*

Together with our distributor, BMG Video, we've sold millions of videos. And along the way, we've acquired a dedicated following who call themselves FIRM Believers. It's even been said that The FIRM has not only changed the direction of the exercise industry but also redefined our national attitude toward health and fitness.

The FIRM was the first fitness program to prove, after extensive research, that aerobics and weight training could (and should) be combined. The result is a supereffective workout that gives *three times the fat loss* of aerobics alone. And, unlike aerobics, The FIRM workout rebuilds the strength (the muscle tissue) that age takes away. It also does a better job of preventing brittle bones and possibly heart disease and stroke as well.

Being "beautiful and youthful" is, in simplest medical terms, nothing more than having a high lean-to-fat body composition ratio. Only The FIRM's "aerobic weight training" simultaneously reverses *both* the muscle loss *and* the fat gain of aging. With The FIRM workout, dramatic exercise results are finally within reach of anyone with a VCR and a willingness to work. In the exercise world that's an historic event.

The FIRM difference has already changed many lives. The FIRM has a hardcore following of perhaps half a million "FIRM Believers," both in our exercise studios and through our videos, who express their gratitude to The FIRM in person, in letter, in e-mail. They report that our workouts not only did wonders for their bodies but in so many cases transformed their general outlook on life as well.

Jane Fonda's office once doubted the authenticity of letters to The FIRM. In 1988, they demanded verification when we reprinted a letter from Maryland in which a FIRM user described a Fonda video as a comparative "joke." We sent a representative sampling of similar letters from FIRM users, and never heard from Fonda's office again.

By conservative estimates, many hundreds of thousands of FIRM users have discovered dramatic results they didn't see with videos by Jane Fonda, Kathy Smith, Richard Simmons, and a hundred other representatives of the reigning "exercise establishment." And due in part to The FIRM's work, women's weight lifting is currently the fastest growing activity in exercise. Even Richard Simmons began promoting weight training—sort of. Simmons has a new companion to his sweatin' tapes: his tonin' tapes with rubber band resistance.

In a 1996 infomercial, Simmons waxed philosophical about his combination of sweatin' and tonin'. As if he had invented the movement, Simmons mused wryly that everyone in fitness seems to be "jumpin' on the bandwagon." (Simmons's tonin' tapes came out years after the key research broke. Welcome aboard.)

For the FIRM Believers and for those of you who have yet to get acquainted with us, we're writing this book to teach you not only our unique approach to exercise, but also the cornerstones of FIRM philosophy: boosting energy levels all day long, staying motivated and upbeat, maximizing nutrition, and reshaping your body while reversing the aging process. We'll draw from the testimonials of FIRM Believers and instructors, including some amazing makeovers, and we'll give you the science behind the exercise and eating plans we recommend—all in accessible, plain English.

We want *FIRM for Life* to serve as your twenty-four-hours-a-day, seven-days-a-week personal trainer—keeping you on the straight and narrow as you move toward your goals. And while The FIRM *fitness* program is essential, FIRM training tips will help you achieve *lifestyle* goals. You'll discover the strong and positive correlation between physical and emotional health and your quality of life. There's no doubt that The FIRM exercise programs work; here we'll prove to you that The FIRM lifestyle is every bit as effective.

DEAR FIRM

"Not only has The FIRM toned my body and helped me lose 'those five stubborn pounds,' it's also helped me improve my posture and chronic back pain. My husband, a former Washington Redskin, used and still uses The FIRM daily to recover from back surgery. He speaks highly of The FIRM and its correct, safe, and effective exercises."

ELIZABETH WYSOCKI, 26,
makeup artist, Falls Church, Virginia

FIRM ROOTS

How in the world did two sisters from South Carolina, without a celebrity spokesperson or a big bankroll, create and bring to market America's top-selling workout videos? We attribute our success to the raw power of a better idea, to our faith that better science eventually wins, and to a family tree ripe with energetic female role models. But most of all, we are grateful to you, The FIRM video users. Thank you for making our work possible. As our work enriches your life, so do your letters enrich ours. Thank you for your many thoughtful letters.

So if you have a workout goal, and you're vaguely ready to commit to it, you've come to the right book! And if you don't have a workout goal yet, this book will give you the motivation you need to commit to a plan! In return, we promise that *you'll see a firmer, shapelier, stronger you in just ten workouts (or less); you'll burn fat three times as fast as with aerobics alone; and, best of all, you'll not be bored!* But first let's tell you a little about ourselves, our background, and how the concept of The FIRM came to be.

GETTING TO KNOW US

We're fifth generation residents of Columbia, South Carolina—baby boomers with a family background that prepared us to fuse dreams with reality and confront the world of the exercise establishment. Our mother, a concert pianist, made her debut at Carnegie Hall when she was nineteen, but gave up a brilliantly promising career to marry and raise four daughters. Our father, a self-employed businessman, was energetic on weekends with all kinds of home projects. We watched him build goat stanchions (to hold the goats in place while we milked them), renovate the goat barn into a bachelor apartment, and build a swimming pool in the backyard for his four daughters. His hobby was calling square dancing, so early on we had an education in group movement to music—one of the cornerstones of The FIRM program.

Ours was a normal fifties father—conservative and ever concerned about the welfare of his girls. Mother, on the other hand, was a risk taker, a bit of a bohemian, and a pioneer who raised us on organic foods decades before it became fashionable. We'll never forget being ridiculed by the other school kids when we took brown bread sandwiches out of our lunch boxes!

A freethinker before her time, Mother read the works of Adele Davis in the mid-1950s. Something "clicked" and she realized that the American "establishment" way of feeding "embalmed" foods to people (especially infants and children) was terrible. Determined to raise a healthy family, she moved us to the country where we were physically active in activities such as growing our own produce, milking goats, making our own butter, and even killing chickens. Having taught us to be unafraid of work, our parents also encouraged us to develop a skill to earn pocket money. (They didn't believe in giving allowances.) Anna taught swimming classes in the backyard, and Cynthia gave piano lessons.

Another great thing about our upbringing was that the house was always filled with artistic talent—cellists, violinists, singers—and project-oriented activity, which fueled our entrepreneurial drive to control our own lives and create a world for others.

At the University of South Carolina, Anna met her future husband and business partner, a young filmmaker named Mark Henriksen. After graduation, Anna and Mark went to Atlanta to edit a documentary film they'd been selected to make, and Cynthia emigrated to Beverly Hills to teach junior high school and subsequently work in commercial real estate. Cynthia always had a head for business and education, and Anna had the passion to create. We were a good team.

Around this time, 1977, Anna was shopping around for a cohesive exercise program. But every gym and studio she tried left her empty and bored, and she knew that boredom was absolute death to any form of exercise: If it bores you, you will quit. It's that simple. Anna claims that her initial motivation for establishing The FIRM was selfish. Since what she wanted and needed didn't exist, she invented a way to train herself that involved synchronization with music and a total body workout.

Since Mark had been lifting weights for a long time, in 1978 he encouraged Anna to bring a pair of dumbbells and ankle weights to her aerobics class. "Without weights, you'll be wasting your time," he advised.

It seemed logical to Mark and Anna that this brand new aerobic weight training combination would produce faster, more dramatic results than any workout class yet invented. Combining aerobics and weights would unite the best of both worlds: (1) the runner's leanness and endurance, and (2) the weight lifter's strength and shapeliness. Great idea. Why not?

Flash-forward seventeen years. In 1995 Dr. Kenneth Cooper (the venerable "father of aerobics") and other luminaries in America's "exercise establishment" revealed their research indicating that aerobics and strength training could be accomplished simultaneously, in one time-efficient workout.

It is ironic that scientific torchbearers such as the Aerobics and Fitness Association of America (AFAA) had previously perpetuated the unscientific belief that aerobic and weight workouts should be done separately. That core belief was based not on scientific research, but on an old gym myth that turned out to be false.

Back in 1978 Anna began using herself as a test subject/guinea pig for the new methodology. Using Mark's recommendations and her own instinctive training, she began selecting and redesigning the basic vocabulary of moves and sequences that would become the core of The FIRM system. As motivation, Anna drew on the usual scientific curiosity, but she also tapped personal vanity—the most common motivator. Anna reasoned that she pursued the same fitness goal as every other woman. Why not use the same motivator? Drawing on her years in the gym, Anna began finding the muscle isolations that she could really feel, within the low-tech/low-boredom parameters of aerobic weight training.

The new workout system results met her high expectations. As predicted, the two-in-one workout produced results. And in 1979 The FIRM's aerobic weight-training classes opened to the public in Charleston, South Carolina. It would be seven years until the first FIRM video was ready for release.

DEAR FIRM

"Hit from behind by a car going one hundred miles per hour, my little pickup truck flew fifty feet in the air and rolled over five times. It took thirty minutes to cut me out with the 'jaws of life.' To the doctors' amazement, my only injuries were a broken arm, broken ribs, and concussions. The medical staff attributed my lack of internal, back, and neck injuries to my good physical condition. I had been doing The FIRM every day. I am fifty-three years old, and whenever I get a physical, they tell me I'm as healthy and fit as a twenty-eight-year-old."

FRANCES B., 53,
Ft. Lauderdale, Florida

PIONEERS IN UNCHARTED TERRITORY

In 1979 (the same year Jane Fonda and Kathy Smith opened less innovative aerobics studios in Los Angeles) Anna, Mark, and Cynthia put The FIRM's system to the test by offering classes in a small Charleston studio—a one-room schoolhouse type of operation—and subsequently in another no-frills space in nearby Columbia. The aerobics establishment immediately tried to blow the whistle on us: When they heard what we were up to, aerobics teachers immediately began warning their students that using weights was *dangerous!* Just why was never made clear.

Let's take a moment to look at how the aerobics explosion began. The dictionary definition of "aerobic" is "occurring in the presence of oxygen"—which applies to any action-oriented workout, from running to swimming, that relies on regularized breathing and that healthfully raises cardiovascular and respiration rates. Americans weren't an exercising population until, in the late sixties, Dr. Kenneth Cooper devised an aerobic fitness program that actually reduced heart attacks in men.

But there was a surprise fringe benefit to Cooper's system: His test group uniformly lost weight. That was the "eureka moment": Aerobics was then taken up by virtually *all* health clubs as a surefire way for women to lose weight.

From the beginning aerobics had problems, although these tended to be overlooked by gyms that were making easy sales from it. Because of the enormous number of repetitions, aerobics could cause injury and certainly produce boredom. Also, although aerobics increased endurance, it couldn't increase strength. To boot, it *primarily* worked only the frontal thigh muscles. High-impact aerobics had its value, but used alone, it couldn't possibly *work and tone* every muscle group in the body the way that The FIRM's system did.

We swam against the high-impact aerobics tide, found our space, and, as in *Field of Dreams,* the customers came. This further agitated the aerobics authorities.

"Women don't want the big, bulging arms and bulky bodies of weight lifters!" cried the detractors. Instructors Anna and Cynthia countered with the truth—that to make the normal female body muscle-bound requires very rare genes, years and years of much heavier lifting than The FIRM's system employed, and (almost always) illegal steroids.

"Okay. Still," they argued, "nothing's better than aerobics for burning fat!" "Not so," the sisters responded. "Our clients have better bodies than the competition's 'aerobics only' instructors!" For fat burning, a combination of weight training and aerobics is far better. Weights add lean muscle. Each pound of muscle burns thirty-five calories a day—calories that would otherwise turn to fat. After thirty-five we lose one-half pound of muscle each year, allowing "middle age spread" to take over. *Only weights restore sleek youthful muscle, while aerobics alone will often cause you to actually lose muscle.*

"But," they went on, "aerobics gives you a natural 'high' that nothing can beat!" Not so, The FIRM countered. Endorphins, the body's natural opiates, are certainly released during an aerobic workout: But aerobic weight training also releases endorphins. Now, it has long been known in weight-lifting circles that a longer-lasting mega-high comes from lifting. Combine aerobics and lifting on a regular basis, and you're actually going to become a generally more upbeat and highly energized person.

Of course they scoffed when we combined the oldest exercise device, the dumbbell, with the newest science, aerobics. Nobody wants a new kid on the block to upset the apple cart of the tried, true, and profitable. But truthfully, the criticism, baseless as it continued to be, was hurtful. Despite the fact that our instructors and clients looked better than the "aerobics only" crowd, the "experts" were blackballing us simply for not conforming to their less effective methods! Here we were, helping people more than established methods could, yet the establishment was treating us like snake-oil salesmen—ones peddling a dangerous elixir at that. Yes, it was frustrating.

DEAR FIRM

"Before The FIRM, I was the stereotypical ninety-eight-pound weakling. Now I am still small, but I feel strong. I have more energy and enjoy life more fully."

PATRICIA KJOLHEDE, 40,
elementary school teacher, Laingsburg, Minnesota

RESULTS YOU CAN SEE

Let's briefly review what made The FIRM methodology so revolutionary—and so threatening to the exercise establishment. Appreciating that aerobics had its benefits, such as burning fat, improving endurance, and strengthening the heart and lungs, we still felt that exercising with that system alone led to overall muscle loss. (Scientific research would verify this point in 1991.) Muscle loss slows metabolism, making it easier to regain fat, and it accelerates aging. We also knew that only weight lifting reversed both major effects of aging: muscle loss and weight gain.

By combining these two disciplines, we were sure we had found a workout plan that would *burn far more fat than* either lifting or aerobics alone—which meant, if we were right, that people would see results fast.

ELIZABETH BASS WORRELL

AGE: 50   PROFESSION: BUSINESS OWNER

Elizabeth decided to become a FIRM instructor in 1992, when she was cast in The FIRM Volume Six video.

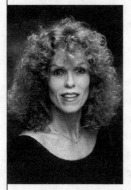

Leading a group through a planned exercise program was a lot harder than Elizabeth had imagined. For the first time, she became fully aware of her personality—weaknesses as well as strengths: "I'm much more sympathetic to the needs of beginners now," she admits.

The FIRM also helped Elizabeth through personal tragedy, the death of her son in 1989. "The grief was overwhelming," she recalls. "Sometimes I'd be working out and could not stop crying, but I held on to my fitness program. Gradually over time, it became better for me. I attribute much of this to the companionship from FIRM Believers. The physical strength I gained during this time also helped me cope with the loss."

Elizabeth makes sure she eats a high-protein, low-fat diet with lots of water, and she doesn't touch sugar or alcohol. She gets her fiber from fruits and vegetables, and she also takes multiple vitamin/mineral and protein supplements because she feels she can't trust her diet to supply all the things she needs. Looking good and feeling good, as well as the exhilaration of the workouts themselves, keep Elizabeth's exercise motivation high.

The FIRM has made Elizabeth believe that you're as young as you feel, and she has a new companion to prove it: "One night," she relates, "I met Richard in a reading bar. He loves the way I look, even though I am almost twenty years older than he is. We share a common interest in bodybuilding—so we have plenty to talk about. I've never been happier!"

ELIZABETH'S TIPS FOR BEGINNERS:

○ That you're building a reserve of strength—both physically and emotionally—is the best reason to stick with a workout program.

○ "You are what you eat" gets truer and truer as you age.

○ Vitamin and mineral supplements guarantee you're getting the best possible nutritional package—I swear by them!

○ You're never too old to grow younger.

When we merged the weight room and the aerobics area in 1979, The FIRM workout studio became the perfect research facility for our clients' benefit and for those who in time would become video customers using inexpensive home gyms. By providing each student with a personal assortment of serious-size dumbbells, The FIRM became *the only low-impact, variable-intensity, total body workout.*

Unlike most other workout facilities, we didn't—and still don't—require clients to sign membership contracts, much less long-term ones. We were aware that the high rate of early dropouts with long contracts was a major source of revenue in conventional gyms. In fact, most gyms make most of their money from dropouts who quit after a few weeks, but keep paying because they signed a contract. Dropout rates are amazingly high: About 75 percent of new gym members drop out by the end of their second month. Many gyms have a hidden agenda secretly *encouraging* newcomers to drop out, thereby enhancing profitability.

The FIRM studio was simply not that kind of place, and its creators were not that kind of people. Everything was (and is) for the good of consumers. Pay by the visit, or by the month. No membership contracts. Unlike conventional gyms, The FIRM has never made money from dropouts. We *lose* money from dropouts. We make money only from those who succeed! If The FIRM workout weren't seriously superior to everything else, we would have disappeared long ago.

We took pains to make our studios as attractive as possible, and our classes relaxed and small. We saw the music synchronization process as key to our program in several ways. We were using it as dancers do—to conquer time by existing in the moment of execution. Because of our music scores, clients could conquer time in the workouts, which, of course, eliminated boredom: You can't be in the moment, totally hyperfocused, and also thinking about the clock.

For each workout, we devised an eclectic music score using techno-pop, dance, reggae, rhythm and blues, Caribbean/tropical, Latin, salsa, African, Celtic, Arabian, cinematic scores, and classical.

Secondly, we took a page from the military drill book and geared our routines to the music's strong and weak beats. You tell people what they're going to do on the weak beat, then have them do the move on the strong beat. That's how the world was different from The FIRM. Most, if not all, exercise classes using music gave the exercisers no advance notice of what was coming next. Imagine an army drill sergeant commanding his unit to turn right—at the very moment of the turn. The result wouldn't be synchronization, but total chaos.

Lastly, again looking to the military, we realized that synchronization bonds people; that's one of the principles of group activity, and it applies to our home exercisers as well. In fact, when we subsequently went to video, the FIRM Believers concept arose because our customers *bonded with the videos.* And music synchronization was in great part responsible for that bond.

Our plan seemed to be on target. Clients always found the classes challenging and innovative. And best of all, they kept coming back!

As for people seeing rapid results, we'd been correct. Compared to any other workout system available then (and now), our program virtually kicked in at once—with clients reporting significant improvements in muscle tone and stamina after only ten classes or fewer. In a poll from 76,000 video purchases, an astonishing 99 percent of the users say that The FIRM is "the most effective workout video I've ever used."

From 1979 to 1985, the pre-video years of testing in our workout studios, more than one million individual workouts were performed by our clients—who represented a statistically meaningful, cross section of average American bodies. Of paramount importance, there were no reports of injury from our new methodology. To this day, with more than three million FIRM videos in circulation, The FIRM's extraordinary safety record stands—as does its record for effectiveness. *The FIRM's guarantee of visible results in ten workouts stands alone.*

Exercise physiologist Dr. Michael Wolf, Ph.D., reviewed The FIRM's first video as not merely safe, but as "super-safe and effective." More than a decade later, Wolf's review has never been seriously challenged. We knew we were on to something that could do people a lot of good, in terms of appearance, health, and self-esteem. What was required was dedication.

Being certified by mainstream groups didn't make sense for us since our exercise program was so different from the general run of gyms and classes. Instead, since 1979, we had been conducting our own rigorous certification program for clients (who successfully auditioned) to become FIRM instructors.

Nevertheless, we continued having trouble with the certifying agencies. When we started The FIRM, we knew we were bending conventional rules about what was considered the right way to work out—but they were right only for *aerobics* teachers! Because typical aerobics classes contained so many repetitions, safety guidelines devised to prevent overuse injuries weren't applicable to FIRM methods. The lower number of repetitions used in The FIRM changes the rules—and requires a different set of safety guidelines.

Just as a playwright might test the draft of a new work by performing it for a live audience, Anna tested drafts of the first FIRM video choreography on clients at The FIRM workout studios. An exercise class is not just the passive recipient of a workout; it can become a participant in crafting the instructor's performance. To the sensitive instructor, the class gives off dozens of nonverbal cues with an expressive variety of looks, hesitations, falterings, smiles, sighs, gasps, and laughter.

During years of teaching, the gifted instructor develops an instinct for reading the clients to know how far to push, when to ease off, and how to build a sequence (both physically and emotionally) with tight music-to-movement synchronization.

The clients also became a source of constant feedback on the effectiveness of the workouts. And more real than any laboratory simulation with recruited test subjects, this was real life itself. Because The FIRM was conceived as a one-room schoolhouse (beginner and advanced clients do the same class, but with different weights), it was the perfect laboratory for developing a workout system for the anonymous, unseen video exercisers we would never actually meet.

As the concept of hiring a personal trainer first spread across America, it occurred to Anna, Mark, and Cynthia that, in a sense, they were involved in creating the ultimate impersonal trainer—a totally self-contained, self-instructing, complete workout system that would reshape the bodies of people they would never see.

The FIRM was born during the early 1980s, at the height of the great aerobics boom. Running was hot. Aerobic dance was hot. It was the Jazzercise age. For an exercise snapshot of the era, rent the video *Perfect*, the 1985 drama about exercise instructor Jamie Lee Curtis and reporter John Travolta.

The aerobics world was very far away from what was happening at The FIRM. In 1983, the Aerobics and Fitness Association of America (AFAA) began selling aerobic certification classes to health club instructors. Today, they are the world's largest trainer of aerobics instructors. In 1986, the International Dance Exercise Association (IDEA) also began selling certification classes for aerobics instructors.

In response to an intense mid-80s media panic over the dubious safety of big doses of high-impact aerobics, a "low-impact" imperative swept over the aerobics world with a vengeance. For aerobic dance, going low impact also meant going low intensity, which also meant low result.

Without intending to, The FIRM workout had already invented low-impact aerobics years earlier, but with wonderfully high intensity—a feat that the aerobics world couldn't accomplish because they didn't use weights.

AFAA and IDEA adopted the role of righteous reformers for exercise safety. Their efforts did help clean up unsafe aerobics classes. But while many bad aerobics practices were rightfully banished, this era also left us with a residue of unreliable, misapplied "safety" ideas that linger on. Chief among them is the faulty notion that low impact is always best. No. As a rule, mixed impact is better/healthier for most of us. (It is superior for preventing brittle bones and for strengthening connective tissue around joints.)

The AFAA/IDEA safety panic had to do with the methods of the aerobics mainstream. The FIRM was already much safer than other methods because it used weights. How could that be? Weights allowed the exerciser to do dozens of exercises that weightless aerobics workouts just couldn't do. With its greater variety of exercises, The FIRM workout spends comparatively little time on any one activity. As a result, The FIRM has almost no chance of causing the overuse injuries that still plague today's aerobics classes and tapes.

In the first Step Reebok® workout video, for example, participants step up and down 369 times—on each leg! Substituting a higher step and optional hand weights, The FIRM's tall step variation requires only about twenty-four repetitions per leg, per workout. With such a low number of reps, overuse injuries just don't happen!

We thought the establishment would come around once they saw our results. No way. We simply couldn't conquer the status quo prejudices—against bodybuilding, for example.

By introducing interval training and alternating activities, we avoided high-repetition injury, as well as boredom. When we reduced the risk of any single component, we felt we'd come upon a new training theory. But the certifying agencies insisted that our use of the word *aerobic* was an unfounded claim.

Having anticipated that the exercise establishment would doubt that The FIRM method was truly aerobic, we had the workout tested in the human performance laboratory at a major university. On both the heart rate test and the oxygen intake test, The FIRM's scores proved that it was indeed solidly aerobic. To drive the point home, we included pictures of the actual testing procedure in *Twenty Questions About Fitness,* The FIRM's fifty-minute educational companion video to the workouts.

But even that didn't seem to convince or deter the establishment. Eleven years after The FIRM premiered on video, we still get the occasional ridiculous review: "May not be aerobic for all levels." Nonsense. When The FIRM's instructors heard that review at a staff meeting, they broke out laughing. "That reviewer obviously never did the tape!" commented one instructor. The entire room nodded in unison.

The establishment just couldn't understand what we were doing because they'd never seen it before. We appreciated that disbelief was natural, almost expected, because of a bias against new methods. But, here again, we couldn't believe their blindness.

Our single consolation is that the vehement outcries against The FIRM have never come from consumers, but from certifying agencies protecting their position as authorities.

"While other institutions were still back in the Stone Age just doing plain aer-obics, I was finding out about the added benefits of using weights, thanks to The FIRM. The FIRM always seems to be on the cutting edge and always chooses methods that don't die."

ANN MODICA, 24,
technical writer, East Meadow, New York

REMOTE CONTROL FITNESS:
HELLO TO VIDEO

Come 1986, we took our next giant step and decided it was now time to "go video." You've got to remember that in the eighties, the VCR (with its accompanying videotapes) was as major a communications break-through as the Internet is today. This time Fonda was out there first, but her workout method was traditional high-impact aerobics—very hard on the body.

No, we didn't have a movie star to showcase our system. No, we didn't have a personal fortune to put into our tapes. But we believed we had what it took to succeed in this brave new market—all with-out leaving home. By this time, Anna and Mark had created two inter-national award-winning film documentaries for . . . well, making boring things interesting. (If ever a perfect résumé for making exercise videos existed, this was it. "Exercise is too boring" is the number one excuse of couch potatoes.) And, having returned to South Carolina to help with the financing for the *film* ventures, Cynthia knew she could raise the money for the *video* venture. Finally, Anna would have to consider herself a fitness innovator—virtually all of our clients not only told us but showed us that.

The team's trio was assembled, the video concepts were completed, but there was the recurring nightmare of raising money. Admittedly, with the first video, we didn't know what we were going to do money-wise, but we had the germ of an idea. The first thing we learned was that going from A to B is really going from A to Z because there are more steps and stops and starts than one can predict.

First, we filmed a pilot starring an instructor named Susan Harris. This was a primitive talent tape, and Susan came out looking like a drowned rat because it was so hot under the lights and she was working out so hard. (We nicknamed the pilot *Torture Tape.*) Anna felt it didn't matter because she believed Susan had "it." We also knew there was no point in going to traditional banks. Real estate financing they understood, but film? You've got nothing there, nothing substantial like a building, until you make the film. Which means that the financing is a highly speculative venture.

So we did the only possible thing: We went to venture capitalists, who were thriving in the eighties. They looked at the *Torture Tape,* then stared at us like we were crazy. We just sat there, trying to read their minds. And Cynthia did! She figured that to these guys, with Jane Fonda's tape just out, fitness was becoming entertainment, which was glamorous, which they liked. They couldn't see through the primitive video to the uniqueness of our program, but they could see that we might be riding a trend. Eventually, we got the money—at a total of 30 percent interest!

Once they gave us the start-up capital, these guys realized they had to give us enough to complete the project, or they'd never recoup their investment. When we paid it back, every cent, we discovered that we were the only good loan they'd ever made.

Armed with the venture capital, we now knew we had no choice. We had to win this one! The program not only had to be superior to all others on the market, but its presentation had to be superior as well! (And because entertainment value is expensive, the videos would have to cost more than all the others on the market.) In the summer of 1984, we began development of the project, from set design to commissioning original music to match the movements. At the same time, we developed choreography and rehearsed Susan Harris (it was the only workout she taught for months!). Finally, during five grueling days in the August heat of 1985, we videotaped the actual workout and information section, and then afterward spent a long nine months editing the show so that the entertainment value would maintain viewer interest as long as possible.

Our first video: *The FIRM: Aerobic Workout with Weights,* later renamed *Body Sculpting Basics,* was the first FIRM workout to achieve classic status when in 1992 *American Health* magazine named it one of the ten best workout videos ever made. We strove to give every customer the working equivalent of a private trainer in the person of The FIRM instructor who led each video.

In the bargain basement land of exercise videos, we were striving for a product as handcrafted and intricately planned and executed as embroidery. And, if planned correctly, the video could become a classic.

For the new video program, The FIRM's method for banishing boredom would be taken to a new level. Mark's architectural talents and cinematic eye gave us a production technique that even other filmmakers couldn't figure out. Anna and Cynthia, from years of teaching experience, knew where the camera should be placed to maintain instructional clarity. They also knew that, for user satisfaction, the music had to be synchronized note by note with the exercises. And, finally, Anna and Mark's film editing instinct for timing—knowing when to move on between exercises and between images—would give the feeling of "being there." The goal was twofold: (1) unmatched fitness results, and (2) award-winning entertainment value to maintain interest.

We knew that most video workouts covertly encourage users to drop out because the tapes are so poorly made and shot. They're so boring, in fact, that it's hard to get through them once. We wanted our customers to come back again and again because they loved and believed in our product, a product that not only worked but had entertainment value as well.

Here again, in more ways than one, we were there first with our flagship video. *Aerobic Workout with Weights* introduced low-impact aerobics long before the exercise industry had a term for it; The FIRM's high-intensity version of low impact is still unsurpassed in effectiveness. Even today, the aerobics establishment is dead set against weight training in groups—which we pioneered.

"Using The FIRM for two and one half years, I continue to see results with every workout. Before, I was convinced that I was just going to have to live with the things I was born with—things I didn't like about my body. But The FIRM has definitely shown me how I'm able to change them."

MARIA S., 27,
bank manager

JOIN THE FIRM: THE DIRECT SELL

Then we hit a snag. When we went to retail video outlets with the tape, they weren't interested. "Where's your celebrity?" they'd ask. We'd tell them, "The show and the results are the celebrities here." They still weren't interested. But if they had a point, so did we. We wanted our clients to be the stars—everyone who followed our routine faithfully and saw results—so why not go directly to them?

Why not take ads in fitness magazines and on cable television describing what was special about The FIRM? Advertise "visible results within ten workouts" and offer customers their money back if the tape doesn't deliver. Why not take a toll-free 800 number and make it easy and inexpensive for interested people to hook up with us? "Reviews Beat Fonda" was an early ad headline grabber. It worked! Sales grew into a steady stream at $49.95 per tape! And every dollar we saved, we put toward our second video because we were being barraged with callers wanting to know when our next tape would be out. Several customers threatened to call us every month or every week until number two appeared.

By the way, the video stores soon came around. It seems that The FIRM was acquiring cult status, and people were not only asking for, but demanding, the tape. We were getting a trickle, then a daily stream of wonderfully encouraging, even inspiring letters, from satisfied customers. The first wave of an eventual hundreds of thousands of FIRM Believers had landed. As the superb reviews and top professional awards for that first video began piling up, it became time to finance our second video.

So we come to the sequel, *Show Me the Money.*

RAISING MONEY FOR RISKY BUSINESS

This time Cynthia decided to go for more traditional fund-raising, but the one banker who had loaned us a small sum for the first FIRM video never seemed to be available when Cynthia called. We had to be extremely creative.

Having been through the rigors of one video, we made some good decisions about the second. We figured we'd built a solid link with the customers, 99 percent of whom were not only satisfied, but desperate for a new video. Bankers didn't understand what was so special about The FIRM. But FIRM users did: They had seen their bodies change. They were the only ones who understood. So we set out to raise video production funds directly from our FIRM customer list. "This will never work," was Mark's response to the plan. "It's our only option," countered Cynthia. "It has to work." Cynthia convinced Mark to compose a heartfelt solicitation flyer that would go to the twenty thousand people who'd bought *FIRM Volume One* and hopefully allow us—in a video first—to presell the second tape months before it would actually be shipped.

We gave ourselves a four-week fund-raising period; in the first week, we received fifty thousand dollars in checks and credit card payments! Incidentally, this pattern was repeated with each ensuing FIRM tape: The FIRM Believers cult had begun!

Then, lo and behold, Cynthia ran into the vanishing banker on an elevator and, since he was a captive audience, he had no choice but to give her an appointment for later that day. So she ran home, put the fifty thousand dollars in a brown paper grocery bag, and set off for the meeting. Presenting him with the paperwork, Cynthia asked for a seventy-five thousand dollar "bridge loan" to begin Volume Two.

He countered with words that meant *no:* "We don't understand the video business."

To which Cynthia replied, "But I bet you understand this!" Slowly, carefully, she reached into the grocery bag and made several piles of the still-unopened envelopes, all of which read "FIRM Volume Two" on the outside. The banker picked them up, scanned the return addresses, and saw that they were from all over the country.

"What's in these?" he asked quizzically.

"Checks for prepaid orders for the video we're going to make," Cynthia replied. "And," she added, dipping back into the grocery bag, "here are the credit card slips."

Once again Cynthia could sense the wheels of his mind starting to turn.

"How much money is this?"

"Well, this is week one of a four-week fund-raising drive. About fifty thousand dollars." It was all Cynthia could do to stop from grinning as the banker mentally multiplied fifty thousand times four.

Then he said the words that meant *yes:* "You don't even need this loan. You need to put this money in a bank."

"You're absolutely right, Jim," Cynthia told him, "I thought you could help me with that."

So we got the loan and learned a lesson: The only time entrepreneurs can expect money from traditional bankers is *when they don't need it.*

That second FIRM workout, released in 1988, defeated Jane Fonda, Kathy Smith, Richard Simmons, and other so-called gurus to capture "Best Health and Fitness Video" awards from *Video Review* and from the prestigious American Film Institute.

A year later, our third FIRM videotape became the first to use the step device on video—years before step aerobics became a hot new trend. By using a higher step as a limited part of the workout, The FIRM step produced even better, faster results, without the "overuse" injuries that plague conventional step aerobics.

Concurrent with that third video's release, *Men's Health* magazine cited scientific studies which found that "moderate-resistance, high-repetition exercise with short rest intervals . . . produces an optimal blood cholesterol change 'for lowering the risk of coronary heart disease.' " This conclusion sees a FIRM-like system as better than straight aerobics (or weight lifting alone) in preventing heart disease—the number one killer.

By 1990, we'd released our fourth FIRM video, featuring shorter aerobic steps, dumbbells, and ankle weights. In the spring of that same year, citing "overwhelming research," the prestigious American College of Sports

Medicine added strength training to its fitness guidelines! Finally, the scientific world was beginning to agree with us.

Our fifth FIRM workout, using both a tall muscle-shaping step and a shorter aerobic step, was released in 1991—the same year that Jane Fonda, admitting business had fallen off, closed her Los Angeles studio.

Also in 1991, aerobics-plus-weights results compared by an independent researcher, YMCA physiologist Wayne Westcott, revealed that the aerobics-plus-weights group yielded 3.1 times the fat loss and added two pounds of muscle, and that the aerobics-only group lost one pound of muscle. That's when we began using the ad claim, "three times the fat loss."

Nineteen ninety-two brought our sixth FIRM tape, which introduced pelvic floor contractions and cast members over sixty years of age. In 1993 came a compilation series of seven "FIRM Parts," which were focused, shorter workouts.

In 1994 and 1995, we presented yet another innovative concept in workouts: cross training, a proven technique for breaking through a stagnant training plateau. In each of these pairs of tapes *(FIRM Strength* and *FIRM Cardio* and *The Tortoise* and *The Hare),* key variables—such as tempo, weight size, and exercise sequencing—are manipulated so that each workout boosts results *when alternated with its companion video.* Used alone, each of these four videos is, of course, a total body workout.

As mentioned, a notable sidebar occurred in 1995 when the father of aerobics, Dr. Ken Cooper, The American College of Sports Medicine, and Nordic Track made the joint announcement that strength training and aerobics need not be segregated into two separate workouts, that both modes of training could be accomplished simultaneously in a single time-efficient workout. Imagine! For nine years The FIRM's central idea, aerobic weight training, had been verified by FIRM video users. We're just wondering how it could have taken the aerobics establishment so long to see it.

In late 1994 we took another giant step. With a burgeoning library of tapes to market, we decided to stop self-distribution and to focus on production. We signed a distribution agreement with a major international company, BMG Video, that would provide FIRM videos with greater marketing clout both here and abroad. This time, the retailers were ready, and so was the public at large! And, Time-Life Video honored FIRM videos by choosing it to comprise its first-ever exercise continuity series.

Research, results, and total dedication to perfecting an inexpensive home workout system is the reason we're number one. We're grateful to have the opportunity to share the message with others. However, even as the research is finally catching up with FIRM methods, there's still plenty of misinformation out there. The source? Ineffective programs promoted by entertainment media, bad science perpetrated by people selling gimmicks, and, perhaps saddest of all, outdated or incorrect science advocated by well-intentioned celebrities.

What a tragedy, when honorable and respectable people flub up! Oprah's bestselling fitness opus, *Make the Connection,* inadvertently promotes out-of-date science. The source? Oprah's well-intentioned but behind-the-times personal trainer, Bob Greene. As mentioned, 1991 was the year of YMCA researcher Wayne Westcott's widely publicized discovery that combining weights and aerobics provides three times the fat loss of aerobics alone. It's understandable that Greene might not be abreast of current minor scientific developments; but Westcott's findings were a major breakthrough that received national attention—five years before Greene's book was published. It's sad that the millions of people who now have read the Oprah/Greene book were misinformed about the critical role that weight lifting plays in weight loss. The table of contents in *Make the Connection* lists Greene's "Ten Steps to a Better Body—and a Better Life." But nowhere in the list is weight lifting even mentioned.

Greene taught Oprah (and now the world) that for fat loss, aerobics is GOOD! Greene started Oprah on hiking, then fast walking and jogging. "What about weights?" asked Katie Couric on NBC's *Today.* For fat loss, says Greene, you should start with aerobics. Weights are good, he says, but only "later on!"

In the Westcott study, exercisers *started out* using weights and aerobics together—and got triple the fat loss of the aerobics-only group *in their first eight weeks!*

While Greene may be a motivating personal coach, his personal belief in starting weights "later on" is contrary to now-proven science.

To Greene's credit, Oprah is now lifting weights. But in light of the research, we believe it's a tragic oversight not to recommend weights for beginners—those who need the encouragement of seeing fast results most desperately! Providing only 30 percent of the fat loss possible by adding weights, Greene's plan for beginners is, unfortunately, a prescription for discouragement.

Greene did spot Oprah's low metabolism. All diet abusers have it: As much as 33 percent (some research says 50 percent) of the weight lost by dieting is not fat, but precious calorie-burning *muscle* tissue! And when dieters regain their lost pounds (as 95 percent do), what they regain is 100 percent fat—and 0 percent muscle! So even when yo-yo dieters return to their exact prediet weights, their percentage of body fat hits an all-time high, and their percentage of lean muscle mass hits an all-time low! Greene thought aerobics would cure Oprah's sagging metabolism. But aerobics boosts metabolism only *during* the walk, and for a limited afterburn period. (For every one hundred calories burned while you exercise, only fifteen additional calories are burned following the workout.) Weight training is the better metabolism booster because it burns extra calories twenty-four hours a day! (One more time: Each pound of added muscle burns an additional thirty-five calories a day—around the clock.) The *ultimate* metabolism booster is aerobics *plus* weights for advanced exercisers *and* for beginners.

Yes, we live in the "Information Age." But it's also the age of *misinformation.* For fitness advice, beware of the TV: On talk show after talk show, Suzanne Somers said that her new Butt Master® would also shape the pectoral muscles under the breasts. Holding the device at chin level, Ms. Somers demonstrated by pulling the gizmo's levers apart. What's wrong with this picture? *Pulling*—as Ms. Somers did—works the upper back. *Pushing* works the chest. If her words *really did* match her actions, her breasts would be on her back!

Selling his "sweatin'" and new "tonin'" videos on a TV shopping channel, Richard Simmons was asked why people needed his "tonin'" tapes. (Using rubber bands, they approximate the resistance training of weights.) "Sometimes when you lose weight, you also lose muscle," said Mr. Simmons. What's wrong with that? It isn't just sometimes that you lose muscle along with fat. It's EVERY time unless you add resistance training! The distinction is critical. Millions of dieters remain obese for life because they don't understand that dieting makes obesity *worse* because it invariably causes muscle loss. Weight training (or enough "tonin'") makes dieting work by causing muscle gain.

Understanding this point clearly would have saved Oprah, for example, from many years of fat-loss failure. On Oprah's show, after her disastrous Optifast® diet in 1988, she bravely wheeled out a wagon containing sixty-seven pounds of animal fat representing her own weight loss. Unfortunately for Oprah, a *true* representation would have included the *many pounds* of muscle that she also lost—nearly one-third of that wagon load! (That lost muscle tissue is the reason Oprah regained all her fat.)

However sincere, charming, and well intentioned, celebrities can be both victims and unknowing perpetrators of weak science. Doctors, the guardians of our health, must also be regarded with some skepticism. Among the bestselling diet books written in recent decades and based on bogus science, at least six were written by doctors.

Depending upon how long ago your doctor went to medical school, his or her entire fitness education may consist of a couple of hours of lecture on the subject. If your doctor is an exerciser, you have the best chance of getting useful information from him or her. But also expect the advice to carry the prejudices and limitations associated with his or her personal exercise preference.

For years we have bemoaned the limitations of the exercise establishment, the lip service to weight training, the misapplication of safety rules, and the failure to confront overuse injury problems with low-impact stepping.

Two factors have kept The FIRM securely on track as we approach the end of its second decade: (1) almost twenty years of using the scientifically correct approach of combining weights and aerobics, and (2) our "living laboratory" of workout studios that filter out all but the best techniques.

Our search for more effective, more interesting methodology never stops. We want to keep our FIRM Believers and ourselves stimulated, committed, and striving every day.

Now we've embarked on a new crusade—to convince beginners and older people that our program isn't only for "hard bodies." We see The

FIRM not only as a series of workout routines but also as the basis for a healthy, active lifestyle, knowing from current scientific findings that strength, flexibility, and wellness can always be increased—whether you're nineteen or ninety.

To that end, our new beginner videos and classes target generations (twenties, thirties, forties, fifties), but certainly can be used by anyone, even if she or he is overweight, out of shape, and/or senior.

Our FIRM CD-ROM will allow home exercisers to create a totally personalized workout tailored to their individual wants and needs.

DEAR FIRM

"The FIRM has drastically changed my opinion of other exercise methods. I will never go back to doing aerobics alone. I have only seen figure changes with The FIRM."

PAULETTE D., 22,
homemaker

CHANGES

For you who are already FIRM Believers, this book will enrich your understanding of our philosophy. To those who are meeting us for the first time, we offer you what you've always wanted—to look better, feel better, and enhance your self-esteem. FIRM Believers know and newcomers will discover that faithfully following our routines will produce remarkable changes, not only in the tone and shape of your body, but in your health, relationships, wardrobe, grooming, activities, food preferences, and cooking style, as well as in your choice of friends and activities. It might interest you to know that our two FIRM studios now offer over 150 classes weekly and are taught by a large number of professional women, including nurses and attorneys—dedicated women who wanted more out of life.

BOYD BRAXTON

AGE: 37   PROFESSION: COMPUTER TECHNICIAN

Trim, dark, and handsome, Boyd—the strong and silent type—is the only male instructor at The FIRM's Columbia studio. He's been teaching classes for six years.

Boyd originally came to The FIRM looking for an efficient way to lose weight. He'd been in a car accident and as a result hadn't been able to

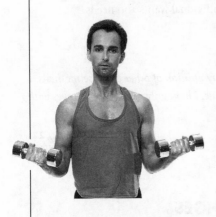

exercise for a long time. As he puts it, "I had gotten big, and I needed to build up my legs. Actually, I went first to the Y and didn't like it. So I went to The FIRM and I've been here ever since. That was in 1991."

In addition to making Boyd a true weight lifter, what has The FIRM done for him? "I have a very stressful job," he explains. "I'm in computers, and my job is pretty demanding, especially in the last year. I think working out and also teaching relieves stress."

Boyd has appeared in several FIRM videos, and claims it's part of the overall fun he experiences at The FIRM. "I enjoy doing the videos. I enjoy teaching. I enjoy the workout and seeing the everyday clients coming back. You know they start out doing five push-ups on their knees, struggling. It's rewarding to see their progress."

And to what does Boyd attribute The FIRM's success rate with clients and video exercisers? His answer is the instructors—who have gone through training, know The FIRM philosophy, and are able to teach it to people. He says he's been to many other gyms where too frequently teachers don't know what they're doing. "They get up there and just do stuff," he comments. "Here, because we're instructed in what we do, The FIRM is different."

BOYD'S TIPS FOR BEGINNERS:

○ Stay focused.

○ Work out consistently—you can't just come in here part of the time.

(continued)

○ Listen to the instructors and follow their leads—they're trained to help you reach your goals.

○ Know what you're doing—if you don't "get it," you won't see progress.

○ Do not expect to come in here and see changes overnight. You must do something for twenty-one days before it becomes a habit.

○ Stay dedicated.

○ Don't try to deprive yourself of all pleasures, but practice moderation in all things and avoid the bad habits that hinder exercise.

FIRM FOR LIFE

Looking back with the wisdom of hindsight, the risks we took look a lot scarier now than they did at the time. Would we do it again? Good question. Perhaps it's a philosophy of life, but we believe that fighting for something worthwhile, struggling against "the system" to create something that changes people's lives for the better, *is* worth the struggle.

And the credit doesn't belong only to us. We share it with every FIRM Believer who has had faith in the program, and the focus and dedication to pursue a vision and make it work. They tell us that The FIRM educated them about their bodies and changed their lives—and that they will be forever grateful.

Next we'd like to explain a little about what awaits you in this book. Chapter 2, FIRM FACTS, will explain in greater detail the science behind the program. It will also discuss the most common questions clients have about exercise. This and every other chapter will be studded with quotes and anecdotes from FIRM Believers' and instructors' profiles.

Chapter 3, FIRM COMMITMENT, deals with setting goals and developing self-confidence through exercise—no matter how improbable this may seem. We'll cut through the excuses for not exercising and provide you with the Keys to Success. Especially entertaining are the Body/Life

Makeover testimonials of FIRM Believers, complete with before and after photographs.

Chapter 4, FIRM FUEL, covers the absolute necessity of proper diet and nutrition. You'll educate yourself about food pyramids, metabolism, food supplements, strategies for lowering the fat in your diet, power foods, the carbohydrate/protein/fat ratio, and much more. We'll give you not only the whys and wherefores but also the menu plans—plus FIRM secrets for never going hungry while staying on the wagon.

Chapter 5, FIRM BODIES, will describe in text and photographs the workouts themselves, emphasizing the importance of variety to avoid boredom. You'll learn the minimum exercise you can do to stay strong and healthy: the Daily Dozen, twelve essential weight-training exercises showing the stop/start positions. Plus breathing, diaphragm contractions, flexibility, and joint rotation—different from aerobic weight training but just as important for stress reduction and relaxation. Plus cardio mini-sweat sessions you can fit into a free moment or two.

Chapter 6, FIRM SPIRITS, will serve to build self-confidence in all areas of your life. After all, you can't just focus on the body and forget about the spirit.

Now that you're looking good, you'll be feeling good, and this chapter will show you how to extend that sense of well-being into your home life, relationships, career, and sense of adventure. The emphasis here is on graceful living, on refining your physical poise and movement in order to stay active, young, healthy, and content.

Chapter 7, FIRM RESOLVE, will review The FIRM Daily Planner, which provides a week's worth of pages that function as a health and workout scheduler, a diet analyzer, a workout inventory, and a personality snapshot. Using these pages as a template, you can go on to create your own journal.

A Glossary of FIRM definitions will fill you in on hot button workout words, dispelling the mystique and making you secure that you know what you're doing.

Our personal journey with The FIRM has certainly been a Herculean effort, but more than that it's been a growth experience, as our studio clients and home exercisers tell us the workouts have been—and as we intend this book to be for you. Begin by accepting the fact that aerobic weight training, in addition to its myriad physical benefits, can be an enormously stabilizing influence, even a safety net, in times of major change—whether the predicament is breaking bad habits, moving to another city, a personal tragedy like Elizabeth Bass Worrell's, a marriage or divorce, childbearing, menopause, or a new job. Why would anybody want to do without it when they don't have to?

Both of us hope that *FIRM for Life* will spark your desire to grow fit, trim, strong, and energized—indefinitely.

Welcome to The FIRM!

CHAPTER 2

FIRM
facts

N ow, get ready for a shock: About half of what you think you know about exercise is *wrong!* In this chapter, you will get a rock-solid grounding in the all-important basic science of exercise. Knowing the basics of how your body works is a great motivator and will take you an incredible distance toward your goal.

DEAR FIRM

"I quit smoking without weight gain!"

KATHRYN L., 29,
association manager, Montgomery, Alabama

WE ARE FOUNTAINS, NOT STATUES

Before trying to change ourselves, let's ask, "What are we?" French existential philosopher Jean Paul Sartre in *Being and Nothingness* divides existence into two states: (1) that which exists "in itself" (material objects such as rocks) and (2) that which exists "for itself" (energies and forces such as lightning bolts, which exist only while in motion). Which are we? Our physical body exists in itself, but as living creatures we exist *primarily* as dynamic energy, force, movement, and action.

We are not like a statue, but like an ever-changing fountain—existing only as long as the force of water pressure sustains it in the air. Like a fountain, our bodies are shaped and sustained, poorly or well, by the quality of the life force supplied by our lifestyles: exercise, food, stress, relaxation, stimulation, and sleep.

The inner universe of your body is unexpectedly dynamic. Every six months, every protein molecule in your body is broken down and replaced. It is estimated that your entire skeleton is completely torn down and rebuilt every two years! Reaching adulthood, we cease "growing"—but never stop rebuilding. Whether you are rebuilt poorly or well depends on you.

DEAR FIRM

"Two years and forty-five pounds ago, I found the best thing going. Only The FIRM lets me build muscle, lose fat, and have fun also! Nothing else even comes close."

STEPHANIE WIGGERS, 28,
college student, Round Rock, Texas

OUR FATE TO BE FAT

Where did your body come from? You inherited it from your tenacious hunter-gatherer ancestors who, according to researchers, burned 2,900 calories a day. Today's average American is a comparative softie, burning just 1,800 calories a day. We were born with an inherited craving for 1,100 a day more than we need!

To burn those 1,100 extra calories, your ancestors did a lot of aerobics as they hunted and gathered—walking or running eleven miles a day, on average, more than we do. (REMEMBER: Running or walking burns almost the same number of calories—about 100 calories per mile, for an adult.) Unwilling/unable to resist our abundant food supply, and unwilling to exercise away the excess calories, the big fat majority of Americans are predictably large and overweight.

The *New York Times* recently reported that, for the first time, overweight Americans outnumber normal Americans: More than half of all Americans are now officially "obese," and it's getting worse. In recent decades, calorie intake has increased by 12 percent. And obesity has increased by 31 percent, with child and adolescent obesity climbing even faster. Experts warn that if obesity continues as it has, everyone in America will be obese by the year 2230. It's an epidemic.

Via evolutionary adaptation, our bodies are designed for coping with (1) scarce food, and (2) a demanding daily workout schedule. (Two hours of very strenuous working out would not equal the 1,100 extra calories burned daily by the hunter-gatherer.)

Suddenly, modern man has reversed both of the circumstances for which evolution designed his body chemistry. We have (1) too many tempting calories, and (2) no need to move or lift. Evolutionary strangers in a strange land, our bodies cannot survive the drastic difference. "Obesity," NBC News recently stated, "is America's biggest health problem." As the process of natural selection continues, the obese are currently being weeded out—dying younger than those who obey the evolutionary mandate to move more and eat less.

EVOLUTION VS. DIETING

It's true that diets don't work if you're talking about a flat-out cure for obesity. *Dieting* meaning "calorie restriction," however, is a necessary *part* of the solution. Researchers found out that dieting doesn't halt obesity because evolution has programmed our bodies with all manner of devious mechanisms to defeat dieting. Why? The hunter-gatherer body we inherited interprets calorie restriction as an emergency warning that famine is coming. Programmed to survive food shortages, your body counters your diet by *increasing* its ability to deposit fat—so that you can wait out the famine.

The more severe your diet, the harder your body fights to hang on to your fat—and make more fat. Going on a fast, even for twenty-four hours, invites disaster. A study on dieting rats (cited by Covert Bailey in *The New Fit or Fat*) illustrates this point: Two groups of rats were put on identical low-calorie diets. One group was further restricted by having to eat all its calories in one big daily meal. After six weeks researchers measured the rat enzymes that control the deposit of fat. The "one meal" group had nearly ten times the amount of fat-producing enzymes as the "nibbler" group!

The "one meal" group had been primed to become megafat producers the moment the diet ended. (After the diet, it took eighteen weeks for enzyme levels of the "one meal" group to return to normal.)

"The FIRM's aerobic weight training gets the job done in half the time!"

CAROLINE PREVOST, 32,
aerobics instructor and personal trainer, Honolulu, Hawaii

HOW DIETS DAMAGE YOU: MUSCLE LOSS

Faced with calorie restriction, your body's most potent fat-saving move is to cannibalize your muscles for fuel. Once oblivious to the distinction between "weight loss" and "fat loss," dieters suffer dearly for not understanding one key fact: As we pointed out earlier when discussing Oprah Winfrey's weight loss, up to one-third of the weight loss from dieting is not fat, but muscle. And that fact is the reason that dieters almost always regain every ounce of lost fat—and more.

Male or female, the body gets its beautiful, youthful shape from having a strong, well-toned muscle system. Having muscle slims down your fat layer because muscle is a very active, ravenous tissue: Each pound of muscle burns thirty-five calories a day, just to stay alive. Just by sitting there, three pounds of muscle burns as many calories as running one mile each day! By comparison, a pound of fat is really dead weight—burning only two calories a day.

After every diet attempt, your body is damaged by muscle loss. And for each pound of muscle you lose, your body burns thirty-five fewer calories each day. (In other words, your metabolism slows.) When you return to eating normally again, you gain weight rapidly because calories you used to burn each day are now being stored as fat. When you gain back all the weight you lost, you are still worse off than before your diet: Assume you lost ten pounds total, comprised of seven pounds of fat and three pounds of muscle. What you gain back is 100 percent pure fat! Although you weigh the same as before your diet, your percentage of body fat is higher than ever. After all that suffering and deprivation, your diet made your obesity *worse*.

That's how the stage is set for a tragic lifetime of yo-yo dieting: After each diet, your body-fat percentage goes higher and higher. Your metabolism sinks lower and lower. Yet every year, 80 percent of the overweight try dieting to lose it. Dieters don't fail because they lack willpower. Dieters fail because evolution defeats them. Do restrict calories and stop yourself from overeating. Do not diet unless you simultaneously lift weights to retain your muscle tissue!

Unfortunately, girls and young women are never told how important it is to have strong muscles. Nobody ever said, "You know, Susie, you would look terrific and feel great if you put on ten pounds of muscle. Let's have a little talk about pumping iron." Times are changing, but most women still don't care about gaining muscle until they find out that after age thirty-five they're losing it at the rate of half a pound a year.

Between the ages of twenty-five and sixty-five, we typically lose 30 to 40 percent of our muscle mass. As the shrinking muscle system consumes fewer and fewer calories, a woman's body-fat percentage typically increases from 25 to 43 percent. A man's body-fat percentage typically increases from 18 to 38 percent. By increasing your body fat and shrinking your muscle system, dieting accelerates your journey from "young and strong" to "old and fat."

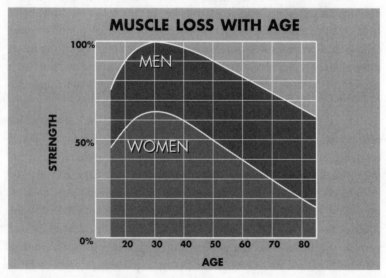

FIVE ESSENTIAL NUMBERS

Worth remembering, these numbers make it easy to make smart choices.

3,500	Calories stored in one pound of FAT.
35	Calories burned daily by one pound of MUSCLE.
2	Calories burned daily by one pound of FAT.
1/2 pound	MUSCLE LOST each year after age thirty-five.
1 1/2 pounds	FAT GAINED each year after age thirty-five.

Armed with these simple numbers, you can understand the inescapable mathematics of aging and obesity. Example: Compared to this date last year, you burned fifteen fewer calories today.

It is said that one can't predict the future, but that's not entirely true. We can, for example, tell you exactly how old you will be in ten years. And unless you intervene (by lifting weights), you will have fifteen more pounds of fat, which you will carry around with five fewer pounds of muscle.

DEAR FIRM

"Since starting The FIRM, I feel healthier. I have been involved in a bone mass density study and my bone mass has increased since adding resistance training—a real benefit for women."

**DEBORAH FREDERICK, 38,
registered nurse, Piermont, New York**

FOREVER YOUNG AND BEAUTIFUL:
PUMPING IRON PAYS

Just as the first wave of science extended our life expectancy, a second wave of science is extending the quality of our now longer lives. In recent years U.S. government research on the prevention of aging has produced dramatic, surprising, encouraging results. What did scientists learn? After completing a massive USDA study on aging, researcher William Evans was

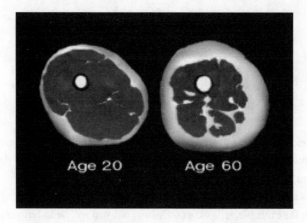

Age 20   Age 60

Aging: A Look Inside
Cross sections of thighs (shown by magnetic imaging) reveal startling muscle loss and fat gain of aging. An athletic twenty-year-old woman is compared to a sedentary sixty-year-old woman. By combining weights and aerobics, The FIRM workout reverses both muscle loss and fat gain.

asked to name the most important single thing one can do to prevent aging. He answered with just two words: "Lift weights."

As the average life span approaches seventy-nine years, most Americans will spend their last twenty years in the "disability zone." Between ages twenty and seventy, inactivity causes us to lose about 30 percent of our strength and 40 percent of our muscle size.

Many of the elderly are forced into nursing homes not because they're sick, but because they are simply too weak to live independently. In one study, one third of sixty-year-old women could not lift ten pounds. It is estimated that one in four people over age sixty-five can't bathe, dress, eat, or get out of bed without help. By age eighty-five, *half* of us can't bathe, dress, eat, or get out of bed without help. In Los Angeles, city planners discovered that one out of four people over age sixty-five cannot make it across a street during a twenty-seven-second green light.

In most cases, weight lifting can delay or prevent the loss of independence.

The medical term for the creeping weakness of aging is "sarcopenia"—Greek for "reduced flesh." Sarcopenia is the accumulated result of losing half a pound of muscle year after year. At any age, weight lifting reverses it.

Earlier researchers had wrongly assumed that the elderly shouldn't lift weights at the same high-intensity level appropriate for younger people. But the results of low-intensity weight work for the elderly were unimpressive. The recent breakthrough began when government researchers tried high-intensity lifting for the elderly—and made amazing progress. At any age, researchers discovered, muscle cells respond to high-intensity weight lifting. In one eight-week study, even women in their nineties tripled their leg strength! (This does not mean that strength gains are quick and easy for the elderly. When muscle strength starts extremely low, even tripling that strength does not make it very strong.)

The bottom line is this: Even late in old age, muscular strength can be regained with serious weight lifting. Starting younger is better. The results of lifting for an entire lifetime are truly astonishing: In one study, weight-lifting "master athletes" in their seventies had the same muscle size and strength as sedentary men in their twenties! Muscle tissue biopsies of older weight lifters likewise resembled the muscle tissue samples from twenty-year-olds. A lifetime of lifting prevented the typical age-related changes found in muscle biopsies of sedentary middle-agers.

In a recent television interview, legendary exercise advocate Jack LaLanne appeared poolside in swimming trunks at age eighty-two. LaLanne's skin looked appropriately crepey (the skin loses elasticity as we age), so one felt that even Jack LaLanne might wear more clothes. But when he suddenly smiled and hit his side chest pose, the audience must have gasped. At age eighty-two, LaLanne still has the beautiful, full musculature of a bodybuilder less than half his age.

"Exercise and temperance," said the Roman poet Cicero, "will preserve something of our youthful vigor, even in old age." Government researchers and Jack LaLanne proved he was absolutely right.

DEBBIE BOYER

AGE: 44   PROFESSION: CRITICAL CARE NURSE

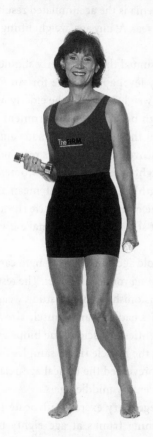

Debbie's memorable smile, distinguished presence, and inner strength and warmth have made her a favorite instructor for the thirteen years she's taught at The FIRM. She's also been a personal trainer for five years.

Unlike many of The FIRM's instructors, Debbie didn't come to the workouts to lose weight. "I've always loved to exercise," she says. "A friend of mine came here all the time, so I took one class and fell in love with it."

Debbie is married to a physician and has two children—a son at West Point and a daughter who just graduated from college on a running scholarship. They are the epitome of a healthy, athletic family.

Since her father died at the age of forty-two, Debbie has long appreciated the need to exercise. She and her family run, play tennis, keep active, and eat well. Although her busy schedule of nursing, instructing, and personal training takes up a lot of her time, Debbie is fortunate in that her family is extremely supportive of her busy schedule.

Debbie has a quiet confidence that makes you trust her instantly. She seems so well balanced, it's difficult to imagine she has problems. "Oh, I'm hyper," she protests. "I'm definitely a Type A personality." That's how Debbie modestly sees herself. Others see a vital woman at the peak of health and fitness, with a boundless store of knowledge, compassion, and energy that people of any age would envy.

(continued)

DEBBIE'S TIPS FOR BEGINNERS:
○ Find a role model; for older people, I'm one. They think, "If she can do it, I can do it!"
○ Set realizable goals: I have a nice body for a forty-four-year-old, but I'll never look twenty-five again.
○ Never forget that exercise makes you feel good about yourself—and it's a great de-stressor!
○ Exercise relieves depression—I never get depressed, I'm always in a good mood.
○ Choose an exercise situation that is like family, not hard-edged and fiercely competitive.
○ Devote your time to living healthy and spending as much time as possible in healthy environments.

NO MORE DANCING GRANNIES, PLEASE

"Endurance training is good," concluded government researchers, "but it won't keep people from getting weak as they get older." Like almost all workout videos, those that successfully target older exercisers are low-impact, low-intensity aerobics videos such as "Dancing Grannies" and Richard Simmons's "Silver Foxes." In light of what researchers now understand about what really does work for older exercisers, one can only say that these video ventures were better than nothing—but not much. For decades, the media has preached the value of endurance training (aka aerobics) for everyone. But clearly what older people need *most* is increased strength and muscle mass. Endurance training provides neither!

Seeing elderly mall walkers, exercise researchers must be filled with ambivalence. Yes, mall walking is indeed "better than nothing," but is that enough? In a three-month study by Larry A. Tucker, Ph.D., professor and director of health promotion at Brigham Young University, the benefits of walking and the benefits of weight lifting on sixty middle-aged women were compared. The weight-lifting group reported nearly twice the "body improvement" of the walking group. Twice is a big difference. Whether you are motivated by (1) the healthy vanity of wanting to look better, or (2) extra years of independent mobility, the clear scientific choice is weight lifting.

People complain that scientific research is subject to sudden contradiction and change, and that they don't know what choices to make amid so much conflicting advice. But the scientific evidence supporting weight lifting is utterly overwhelming and without contradiction. "Strength training," reports the *Harvard Health Letter*, "is the closest thing there is to a fountain of youth."

Having read the litany of facts already presented, you really have only two choices: (1) start lifting, or (2) live in denial regarding your later years.

Composing what could have been a motto for the "wellness movement," Francis Bacon once wrote, "Knowledge itself is power. Chiefly the mold of a man's fortune is in his own hands." Knowledge of weight lifting is so powerful it can change your entire life. Researchers in aging prevention lament that doctors are years away from having an adequate understanding of the subject.

With the discovery of weight lifting's medical benefits comes the realization that you can take charge of your body. You can't get a doctor to lift the weights for you. It is the mandatory do-it-yourself nature of weight training that makes it an appealingly democratic leveler of humanity: Rich or poor, young or old, if you want the benefits, you have to do the lifting yourself.

At The FIRM, it is inspiring to see older people lifting. Few things are as life-affirming as a good workout. The age factor adds another level of poignancy—recognition of the continuity of life. In the past most gym populations were so utterly youth-dominated that being older generally meant over thirty-five. Though slowly, the median age in the gym world is moving up to include those who benefit most from weight lifting—the elderly.

DEAR FIRM

"I did aerobics, Nautilus, racquetball, and step classes for seven years . . . and after one year with The FIRM, I had more results than in all the seven years. My husband tells me I look better than at any time in our marriage, and he tells me all the time."

CYNTHIA C. BLACKBURN, 41,
wife, mother, and partner in husband's business,
Kernersville, North Carolina

MYTH NUMBER ONE:
WEIGHTS WILL GIVE WOMEN BIG MUSCLES

We suspect this myth endures for two reasons: (1) People haven't been properly educated and/or aren't willing to use their common sense; and (2) Women simply *want* to believe it's true so as to give themselves an excuse for not exercising. Ask anyone who subscribes to this myth if they or their friends have ever known a woman who developed oversized muscles from weight lifting. They will admit they haven't; yet the myth lives on! Go figure.

The reality is that for both sexes, only weight lifting can boost metabolism around the clock. (The post-exercise afterburn from aerobics also boosts metabolism, but the effect is comparatively brief.) Only weights can dramatically reverse the muscle-to-fat body composition shift of aging. And only weights can make you look dramatically slimmer, younger, and more beautiful—at any age.

Only about two percent of women have the rare body chemistry that would make large muscles possible, and only after years of lifting very heavy weights—much heavier than the five-, eight-, ten- and fifteen-pound dumbbells used in The FIRM workouts. The truth is women can increase strength by 44 percent without increasing muscle size.

As the public is increasingly aware, virtually all female bodybuilders achieve their extreme muscularity by using illegal steroids. Chemically speaking, the rest of us are fundamentally different from the drug-enhanced pro female bodybuilders.

Women who have never been in a gym fear getting huge muscles. But women who do lift weights soon learn the truth: Increasing muscle size is difficult enough for men (who want big muscles), but even more difficult for women. That's because muscle growth is controlled by the male hormone *testosterone,* and women have only one-tenth as much as men. That's why men have to shave in the morning and women don't, and why men use heavier weights and gain more muscle than women—even with the same workout.

By using steroids, a woman can have a testosterone level that's higher than the average man's! For women, steroids bring serious health risks as well as a peculiar masculinization of secondary body characteristics: When asked about the deep voices of the East German 1976 Olympic team's female swimmers, the coach replied evasively, "We have come here to swim, not sing."

Our male clients enjoy adding muscle because men have always known that it makes them more youthful and "manly." But for women it is a surprisingly modern rediscovery that the same techniques make women more youthful and "womanly."

MYTH NUMBER TWO: "MUSCLES TURN TO FLAB" IF YOU QUIT LIFTING

If you stop lifting weights, muscles atrophy just as they do when one ages. Muscles slowly shrink in size and strength as muscle tissue is carried away by the bloodstream. Unused muscles don't change into anything.

DEAR FIRM

"If anyone had told me fourteen years ago when I was diagnosed with arthritis that I would be lifting weights, dancing, and stepping, I would have told them they were nuts. Now I'm stronger than a healthy eighteen-year-old. The FIRM has helped stop the degeneration in my joints. Thanks!"

TERESA DEREGGE, 38,
writer, Dallas, Texas

HOW WEIGHTS WORK

The goal of weight training is to totally exhaust the target muscle, thereby stimulating it to grow back just a bit stronger during the rest period between workouts. The technique is called *progressive overload*. We first learned about this technique in an early childhood story about a farmer who lifted a calf every day as it grew. And eventually, the farmer could lift the fully grown cow.

That story is based on a real historical figure named Milo, a strength athlete, born in southern Italy circa 558 B.C. Milo trained by shouldering a young cow and carrying it the length of the stadium at Olympia, until the cow was four years old. For this, Milo is often credited with inventing progressive overload and the first barbell—a cow.

In modern weight workouts, the goal is to completely exhaust one muscle group, then do the same to the next muscle group, and so forth until the entire body (or sometimes half of it) has been worked. Bodybuilders typically do each exercise about ten times in a row. In weight lifting lingo, this becomes "ten *repetitions*" (or "ten *reps*") in one *"set"* (a series of reps done without stopping). For each exercise, bodybuilders typically perform "three sets of ten reps," with rest periods of about one minute between sets.

A hybrid of weight lifting and aerobics, The FIRM workout combines the benefits of *both* types of training by using more reps and lighter weights than standard bodybuilding. The FIRM uses the classic bodybuilding isolation exercises, but in new combinations and synchronized to music.

To succeed at weight lifting, you need to know what happens inside your muscles. Each of your muscles is made up of bundles within bundles of individual muscle fibers. When you exercise, each individual fiber either contracts totally or not at all.

The heavier the dumbbell, the more fibers contract to overcome it. The closer you come to exhausting all the fibers, the faster you'll see results.

As you reach the point of "muscle failure," you'll feel "the burn" (the healthy pain of exercise) in the belly of the muscle. The burn grows as *lactic acid* (a waste product of exercise) builds in the muscle, and stops when you stop the exercise.

MYTH NUMBER THREE: NO PAIN, NO GAIN

Endless arguments are held on whether or not exercise should "hurt." The answer is yes and no. Yes to the burn pain, and no to the pain of injury. (The Greeks had six words for different kinds of love; we need at least two for different kinds of pain.)

Unlike the burn, injury causes a sharp pain and usually results from insufficient warm-up, or "jerking" the weights.

It is not necessary to exercise to the burn point to get results, but it will give you maximum results in minimum time. Since fast results make the difference between a program you will stick with and one you will quit, we recommend that you eventually go for the burn.

You will, however, have to work to at least 60 percent of muscle failure to even begin to get results. Many common exercises don't work without weights because you can't get to 60 percent of maximum by flapping your arms!

DEAR FIRM

"The FIRM's aerobic weight training methods are especially effective because they build muscular endurance. I feel better exercising regularly and have lots of energy. I've had three children and I'm happy to report I'm still a size 4–6!"

LYNN E. KAVCSAK, 36,
academic, Raleigh, North Carolina

WHAT'S WRONG WITH AEROBICS?

On the Internet, aerobic exercisers and weight lifters had so much disagreement over goals and methods that they broke off into separate discussion groups. The FIRM is one of the few places that both aerobics and lifting coexist in harmony.

"Is Aerobics Dead?" asked a headline in *Women's Sports and Fitness.* Health club aerobics classes, noted the article, have been largely replaced by body sculpting classes. Father of aerobics Dr. Kenneth Cooper recently noted that Americans' participation in aerobics has dropped from nearly 60 percent a decade ago to closer to 30 percent today. In the same decade that participation in aerobics fizzled to half its previous level, the fastest-growing exercise boom became women who lift weights. According to a study by the Fitness Products Council, the number of women lifting weights *quadrupled* between 1987 and 1995. For men and women combined, weight lifting is now more popular than walking: 18.6 million lifters vs. 17.2 million walkers! Americans are exercising smarter.

During the big 1980s aerobics boom, the benefits of aerobics had been grossly oversold by both the fitness establishment and by the mainstream media. Aerobics, promised the media, would save us from our fat cells. The myth of aerobics benefits finally began to crumble in 1990, when the venerable American College of Sports Medicine (ACSM) added weight training to its exercise recommendations. "It seemed like during the aerobics boom, we went to one extreme," admitted exercise physiologist Michael L. Pollock, chairman of the ACSM recommendations committee, "probably because there was a lack of data on weight training. Now the research is overwhelming." And that was *before* the recent research on weights and aging prevention.

The next blow to aerobics came in 1991 when researcher Wayne Westcott compared fat loss of aerobic exercisers with fat loss of exercisers who did both aerobics *and weights.* Westcott's widely publicized results showed *three times the fat loss with the weights/aerobics combination exercisers.*

Coincidentally just one month after this research appeared, Jane Fonda admitted that business was down at her famous Beverly Hills aerobics studio and closed its doors. In the final analysis, aerobics is a brilliant concept and a wonderful *part* of a workout, but clearly not the most important part. Exercise is a stool with three legs: strength, flexibility, and aerobics. Remove any one element, and the stool falls. Standing alone, aerobic results are simply not as dramatic as experts once claimed.

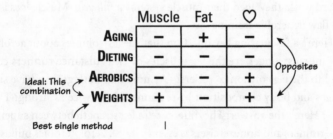

This nifty chart makes it easy to understand the various effects that aerobics, weights, dieting, and aging have on your body: (1) your muscles, (2) your fat layer, and (3) your heart. In the simplest plus-or-minus terms, the chart shows the positives and negatives of the methods used to control fat.

As the chart indicates, every consequence of aging is bad: less muscle, more fat, and less heart muscle. (As your heart muscle shrinks with age, your aerobic fitness drops about 15 percent per decade.) Except for its ability to remove fat (at least temporarily), dieting has the same bad effects as aging: less muscle, and less heart muscle.

It is not a new discovery that like aging, dieting causes the loss of heart muscle. In 1976, Dr. Robert Linn tried to remedy the problem of dieters' muscle loss with *The Last Chance Diet,* which introduced the "protein-sparing modified fast." Dieters were allowed three hundred calories of a nasty-tasting liquid protein mixture, intended to keep them from cannibalizing their own muscle tissue for fuel. But in 1977, more than fifty people died on liquid protein diets. Autopsies revealed atrophy (shrinkage) of the heart, one of many muscles the body consumes during times of starvation. The same phenomenon leads to heart attacks in victims of anorexia.

Aerobic exercise is the champion at strengthening the heart muscle. Aerobics also burns calories. And in significant doses, aerobics can bring about a euphoria ("runners' high") caused by the body's release of natural morphine-like substances called endorphins.

Unfortunately, aerobics has a dirty little secret: Except in the heart, *aerobics causes muscle loss.* In other words, aerobics *ages your muscle system.* A two-month study of stationary bicyclers revealed that the subjects lost three pounds of fat, but also lost a half pound of muscle. With *two months* of hard work, they aged their muscle systems *a full year.* Muscle loss is the fatal flaw in aerobic training.

Here's a fascinating key question that speaks volumes about aerobics: How much stronger are the leg muscles of elite, distance runners compared to the legs of nonexercisers? (Assume that both groups have similar ages and body composition.) Are runners' legs twice as strong? Three times? Here's the answer: The difference in leg strength between superdistance runners and nonexercisers is essentially . . . zero! Aerobics builds endurance, not strength. (The heart is the *only* muscle made stronger by aerobics.)

Aerobics does not build strength, but it does not follow that strength training does not improve aerobic capacity. It does. Research shows that exercisers who are given only strength-training exercises (and no aerobic work) will improve in both strength *and* aerobic endurance! In fact, strength training makes an excellent preparation for aerobics classes, because executing an aerobic routine without clumsiness requires strength—which aerobics won't develop.

As with dieting, aerobics backfires when you stop (because of lost muscle), eventually causing fat gain.

Weight lifting is, as the chart indicates, the perfect antidote for aging. Everything that aging does, weights can undo: replace muscle tissue, remove fat, and even help rebuild heart muscle.

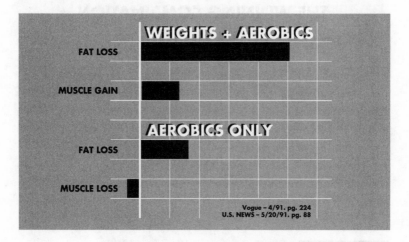

Vogue – 4/91. pg. 224
U.S. NEWS – 5/20/91. pg. 88

REVERSING BONE LOSS

Weight training is also the most effective way to prevent brittle bones. Osteoporosis is extremely common and the effects are tragic. *Prevention* magazine reported that as many as one quarter of those who sustain a hip fracture over the age of fifty die within the year, and research at Tufts University found that among the elderly, broken bones are the leading cause of accidental death. Compared to breast cancer, four times as many women will suffer from osteoporosis: One in two women over fifty (and one in four men) will break a bone due to osteoporosis.

People forget that bones are alive. Like muscles, bones grow stronger in response to the stress of weight lifting. Just as the bone in a professional tennis player's racquet arm grows thicker and stronger than his other arm, your bones grow stronger with weight lifting.

Walking is sometimes recommended for the prevention of osteoporosis, but it is much less effective than weight lifting. We're always puzzled when we see walking prescribed for osteoporosis prevention: Studies show that women who walk at least a mile a day lose bone more slowly than nonwalkers (which is good), but they are still losing bone. Only weight training can *increase* bone mass—even in the elderly.

THE WINNING COMBINATION

Weight lifting not only makes dieting and aerobics safe (by preventing muscle loss), it also causes fat loss in two ways: (1) you burn extra calories while you lift, and (2) each pound of added muscle burns thirty-five calories a day. Adding just three pounds of muscle to your body burns as many calories as running a mile a day—and burns off an extra pound of fat each month. (When you're not exercising, muscle burns an impressive mix of 70 percent fat and 30 percent glycogen.)

The absolute fastest fitness results come from combining all three fitness activities in this order of priority: (1) weights, (2) aerobics, and (3) dieting.

DEAR FIRM

"I have a ten-month-old son, and I live on the third floor. Now I can carry him up the stairs with no problem. I feel that without The FIRM I could never be in the shape I'm in now."

JENNIFER FROST, 25,
health services, Quincy, Massachusetts

EVALUATING EXERCISE METHODS

Exercise gizmos that advertise a very high number of calories burned per workout (". . . burns up to 750 calories per workout!") have very little chance of working well for you. The claim may be true: Somewhere on

Earth, there may be a super athlete who can burn that many calories in a workout with this device. But you cannot. Not with *any* workout!

Furthermore, any product that boasts about the huge number of calories it burns is almost certain to be a strictly aerobic product, which means it provides only one third the fat loss possible with a weights/aerobics combination. Advertising the high number of calories something burns panders to the popular myth that exercise works simply by burning calories, thus subtracting them from daily calorie intake.

The true measure of a workout's potential results would be (1) calories burned, plus (2) new muscle added. But arriving at a meaningful number to represent these two elements strains the limits of objective testing. (Objective research can tell you how much muscle was added, but not whether new muscle is distributed artistically.)

One common method for determining a workout's potential for cardiorespiratory enhancement is whether or not it burns two hundred or more calories per session. In university tests of The FIRM's complete total-body workout videos, even the very unmotivated test subjects recruited by the university exceeded that number.

University tests also verified that The FIRM's use of variable weight sizes makes each workout appropriately easy for the beginners, or tough for the advanced. With The FIRM, advanced/motivated exercisers can easily burn more than twice the number of calories burned by beginners using the same workout. Beginner or advanced, only The FIRM can hit your desired level of challenge precisely.

In an interesting study of ten people who claimed that they were absolutely unable to lose fat, no matter what, the subjects were asked how many calories they burned with daily exercise. Thinking they worked off 1,022 calories a day with exercise, they actually burned off only 771 calories—just 75 percent of what they believed.

The study also showed that they underestimated the number of calories they ate. Guessing they consumed only 1,028 calories a day, they actually consumed 2,081 calories a day—more than twice as much! Subtracting calories they thought they burned from calories they thought they ate, these people apparently believed they survived on six calories a day—without losing weight! With just six calories to burn, you would be stone dead within ten minutes.

AEROBIC PULSE CHECK IS OUT

While exercisers may not correctly estimate calories burned or consumed, they can estimate accurately the intensity of their exercise.

It may sound like a strangely unscientific idea, but it's true: Exercisers' *opinions* about how hard they're working are more reliable than the old 1980s method of counting heartbeats to determine exercise intensity! The superior modern method uses the "Rate of Perceived Exertion" (RPE) scale:

Here's how the scale works: During your workout, just ask yourself, "How hard am I working right now?" If your answer is fairly light, somewhat hard, or hard, you know you're in the lower, middle, or upper part of your aerobic zone. It's that easy.

RATE OF PERCEIVED EXERTION SCALE

6	EXTREMELY LIGHT	When you're in this zone, it doesn't feel like exercise—and it's not.
7		
8	VERY LIGHT	Not really "working" yet, this zone is only for the warm-up or cool-down.
9		
10	FAIRLY LIGHT	
11		Your Aerobic Zone: The low end feels easy, but still burns calories.
12	SOMEWHAT HARD	Around 13, you're starting to sweat.
13		Around 15, you're dripping faster and starting to have trouble carrying on a conversation.
14	HARD	
15		
16	VERY HARD	
17		Above your Aerobic Zone: This level is for competitive athletes. Your breathing is labored, you can't talk, and your muscles are burning.
18	EXTREMELY HARD	
19		
20		

Most of the old aerobic prescription still holds: Aerobics should be performed at least three times a week, with at least twenty minutes per workout spent in the aerobic zone. Researchers updated the formula when they learned that the twenty aerobic minutes need not be continuous: Two ten-minute sessions during the day are just as good. (Any number of sessions will work, as long as you spend a total of twenty minutes in your aerobic zone.)

CAN LOW-INTENSITY AEROBICS BURN MORE FAT?

Old myths die hard. It was once believed that for fat loss, longer low-intensity workouts were better than shorter high-intensity workouts. The notion that a low-sweat/no-sweat workout works best is understandably seductive. But like most bad ideas, this theory was based on a half truth.

Low-intensity aerobics does indeed burn *a higher percentage of fat* than high-intensity aerobics. In one study, for example, a half-hour *walk* burned 240 calories—40 percent from fat (96 fat calories). A half-hour *run* burned 450 calories—but only 25 percent from fat (112 fat calories). The runner burned only 16 fat calories more than the walker. But extend the half-hour walk by just four minutes, and the walker would burn *more* fat calories than the runner!

The fallacy in all this is that fat loss does not equal merely the fat calories burned during the workout. There's more to it. The *nonfat* calories you burn also count. (These calories come from glycogen, the sugar that your muscles burn.) It is believed that much of the fat loss from exercise comes *after* the workout, when your body raids its fat stores to replace lost calories. So running does indeed cause greater fat loss than walking. And as you already know, running plus weight training is three times better yet.

DEAR FIRM

"I'm asthmatic and using The FIRM helped build up my lung capacity so that I can run without an asthma attack. The FIRM has also helped my legs, so I can get up a huge hill by our home without getting off the bike and walking."

LANA A. EPISCOPO, 24,
homemaker, accountant for family business, Indian River, Michigan

TARA JUDGE

AGE: 27
PROFESSION: EARNING A GRADUATE DEGREE IN APPLIED HISTORY; WORKS ON FIRM VIDEO PRODUCTIONS; PERSONAL TRAINS AS WELL AS INSTRUCTS

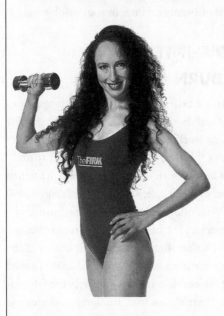

A veteran of dance and fitness classes, Tara started attending The FIRM after college and discovered she wasn't as strong as she thought she was. "I was almost immediately hooked," she explains, "because the classes gave me both the movement I longed for and the strength training I needed."

Since she's been teaching, she feels she's become stronger (especially in the upper body) and more defined and that she has put on a good amount of lean muscle. She's also become a stronger person inside. "I've been shy for most of my life," she confesses, "but The FIRM has made me more confident and outspoken. I've been able to conquer a lot of fears I once had. I'm less inclined to let someone walk all over me. I guess you could say that I've finally begun to develop a backbone."

Tara adds that "teaching at The FIRM has made me more outgoing and has therefore improved the quality of my relationships."

As someone who once suffered from lack of confidence, Tara has emerged a confident and outgoing woman, who can admit, "I'm a pretty happy person. I wish to always be this happy."

(continued)

TARA'S TIPS FOR BEGINNERS:
○ Be well-rounded: Make time for work, play, family, healthy eating, and, of course, exercise.
○ Take it slow at first: Give up or cut down on vices one at a time.
○ If you're completely inactive, get out and walk a few times a week or take a beginner's class.
○ Gradually increase your activity level and intensity as you become stronger.
○ Don't let a setback ruin all that you've accomplished (in other words, don't beat yourself up over a slip).
○ Challenge is part of the shape-up process, whether it's getting a well-toned body or going back to school for another degree: Embrace it!

HOW WILL YOU LOOK
WHEN YOU GET INTO SHAPE?

Soon you'll see muscle tone. A toned muscle is like a fresh piece of fruit—firm, juicy, and alive. Untoned muscles are flat and shapeless.

Even before your scales say you've lost a pound, friends will ask if you've lost weight, because toned muscles give shape to the fat layer on top. Even as you lose fat, gain muscle, and look slimmer, you may weigh the same because muscle is more dense than fat. (Pound for pound, muscle takes up about 75 percent as much space as fat.) Trust your mirror, not your scales.

When your muscles are toned and your fat layer is reduced, you then have muscle definition. For men and women, muscle definition is beautiful and irresistibly sexy. As the pattern of muscles begins to show, the body takes on a sculptural quality that makes you want to touch it.

Muscle development from sports is sport specific: Only the muscles used in the sport are toned. But weight training can scientifically develop *all* the muscles.

The effect is dazzling. Aristotle noted that the ancient Greek pentathletes were the most beautiful creatures in the world because five different sports gave them all-over muscle definition. (Since the ancient Olympics were held entirely in the nude, all-over muscle definition was a doubly impressive sight.) Weight training creates the same effect in much less time than becoming a pentathlete.

Just as curiosity killed the cat, impatience is what kills the beginning exerciser. Don't try to lose more than two pounds a week, even though you're being smart by combining diet and exercise. Exercise makes dieting easier because it reduces appetite.

Women's fat deposits appear in a variety of places: upper arms, abdomen, buttocks, and thighs. Spot reducing is a fraud. Whatever exercises you do, fat deposits come off in the reverse order that they arrived: Last hired, first fired. Men's fat deposits are more centralized on the middle abdomen.

Regarding the dimpled fat called cellulite, avoid special exercises, books, creams, scrubbers, and diets sold to remove it. It's only fat, and is removed with exercise and diet. Cellulite's distinctive puckered look comes from the webwork of connective tissue that holds the fat deposit together just beneath the skin. Because women's skin tends to be thinner, cellulite shows more in women than men. (A bestselling book on cellulite once claimed that it comes from eating modern processed food. Not true. Nineteenth-century nude photography reveals plenty of cellulite.)

DEAR FIRM

"My doctor wanted to prescribe antidepression medication. Since I have been exercising with The FIRM for about four and a half weeks, my moods have improved, and I don't think medication will be necessary."

CATHERINE KUEHN, 28,
graduate student and teacher, Miami, Florida

GET STARTED NOW!

This is *the* most important part. Just as you wouldn't take one violin lesson and expect to play "The Flight of the Bumblebee," don't expect to do the entire workout your first time. Any workout video you can do well the first time is a waste. No challenge, no progress. Remember that exercise is based on progressive overload. Easy exercise is *no* exercise!

In the beginning, don't try to prove anything to anyone—especially to yourself. Do a little of each exercise, but coast through most of the workout. You won't know until the next day whether or not you did too much. For many, their first workout is also their last. They get so sore twenty-four hours later that they feel as if they've been run over by a truck.

Researchers don't know precisely why beginners have next-day soreness, but these four rules for beginners will prevent it:

1. The first day, push yourself only about half as hard as you think you can on any exercise.
2. Use little or no weight the first week.
3. Back off if anything starts to hurt, or if muscles start to tremble.
4. For safety, do the first and last tunes (the warm-up and cool-down) every time you work out.

If you're just a bit sore twenty-four hours after a workout, you're proceeding at the right pace. This doesn't mean your early workouts won't be challenging. Concentrate on learning good form. Don't rush it. Impatience is the prime cause of failure.

It takes about three weeks to break in your body so that you don't get sore anymore. When you make it, you have accomplished something major. Making it through those first three weeks can change your life forever.

Coming off years of inactivity can seem very tough. About ten minutes into your workout, a little demon will tell you to quit. *Don't listen!* Hold on to the image of a sound mind in a sound body.

The amazing human body can survive under very adverse circumstances—junk-food vending machines and no exercise. But for us to thrive and participate in the joy of life, the body's complex mechanisms must have a variety of nutrients and intense physical stimuli. But don't try to be instantly perfect. Radical conversions almost never succeed. Do take the immediate big step of committing to a workout schedule.

Regarding other lifestyle factors, just keep asking yourself if you're doing better this week than last. As long as the answer is yes, your mirror will supply the psychological reinforcement you need to keep moving forward.

CHAPTER 3

FIRM
commitment

We're not here to tell you that getting motivated is a piece of cake. It's rough, very rough, but we've seen again and again that the payoff makes all the struggle worthwhile.

Once, when Cynthia was working in real estate and struggling with it, she forced herself to write, "I can see myself making cold calls and enjoying it." Of course she hated the job, but she had to go in and do it. If she wasn't busy with actual work, she had to make those detestable cold calls—sometimes for two hours, sometimes for eight to ten hours a day. Yes, people continually yelled at her and hung up. But the point is, she did it! And she got results. The success from that tenacity formed a basis for tackling even larger projects. Which is to say there are simply no magic bullets for realizing goals or fulfilling obligations; they're processes that you have to work through.

ARE YOU UP FOR IT?

In the same vein, there's no doubt that following through with an exercise program—especially if you're doing it at home with only yourself to report to—requires a large measure of enterprise, dedication, and resolve.

You visualize a goal, you vow to achieve it, you're willing to discipline yourself for it, you work on focus and commitment, and you build up the drive to keep going through the early rounds until you see results.

That The FIRM shows you those results so quickly is a major motivational plus, as is the compelling nature of the videos, but you still must develop commitment within yourself. Is it a breeze? No. Is it worth digging deep into your nature and coming up with a mental strength you didn't know you had? Ask any FIRM Believer whose life has been transformed by doing just that.

Before we get to the fundamentals of commitment, let's go through the most common excuses people use for *not* working out, then shoot them down, one by one. It's important to recognize these traps and to remember that you can avoid them if you're totally honest with yourself.

DEAR FIRM

"As I grow older, my body gets better and better. I'm even losing dress sizes. All of my peers are going in the opposite direction!"

**HILARY WATSON, 29,
banker, Old Greenwich, Connecticut**

THE TOP TEN ALL-TIME EXERCISE COP-OUTS

1. *I'll exercise only if I have to.* Oh, please! Are you really going to wait until *after* the heart attack? Until you break up a relationship and are looking for a new partner? Until you've gained twenty pounds, don't fit into your clothes, and feel miserable?

Doesn't it make more sense to start today when no major trauma looms on the horizon? That way, you'll be conditioned for change when it occurs, and you'll even avoid many health catastrophes by putting your body in the best shape possible. And with the added strength and energy The FIRM workout provides, you'll be better prepared to deal with whatever unexpected events life hurls at you.

2. *I don't have enough time.* Shame on you! You have time to watch television, go to the movies, hang out with office friends after work—and you're seriously telling us you can't spare four or five hours a week for an activity that has long-term payoffs and multiple satisfactions?

This is all about priorities and what's really important to you. The benefits of exercise are so great that they're worth reordering your schedule. If you're serious about shaping up, you'll find the time somehow, somewhere.

For instance, if you have to get up an hour earlier to do the workout, you'll start the day feeling warmed up, fit, and energized.

If you have to put an hour aside at the end of the day, you'll work off accumulated stress and anxiety and end up feeling refreshed.

If you're home during the day, give up one soap opera, take advantage of the kids being at school or the baby napping, or work out while the laundry is in the machine. Do a tape, ride the exercise bike, use a machine, whatever you prefer.

Give up a lunch hour with chums to go to the gym or, better yet, have them go with you. If you've got gym facilities, or even a VCR in the office, do a tape alone or with others.

Make early weekend mornings your private time to walk, jog, work out, swim—or find another early bird who'd be the perfect tennis partner.

Replace compulsive shopping trips to the mall with the exercise of your choice. Not only will you save money, but you'll look better in anything you try on.

Cut down on "Happy Hours" and use after-office time more healthfully; when you do go out with friends, you'll be in better shape—physically *and* emotionally.

Bottom line: The good news about exercise is that the more time you put in, the more it gives back. Work out now, have more energy later. When you make fitness a priority, you'll be able to do more things in life with less exertion—and you'll look a lot better doing them. For instance, you'll sleep more deeply and arise more rested, although your actual hours at rest are fewer. You'll have better mental focus and get more accomplished in less time. Pretty good deal, right?

3. *I'll always look like the rest of my family.* Many, many people see hereditary similarities between themselves and others in their family and feel discouraged. Frankly, it's no excuse. The quest for a well-proportioned physique shouldn't be compromised by what you exaggeratedly regard as *genetic doom.*

If you look at pictures of your relatives from the turn of the century, they're shorter and rounder. Better nutrition has made people today taller and healthier. We now have the knowledge and technology at our disposal to reshape our bodies, slow down the aging process, and be healthier. Use it; don't abuse genetics as a lame excuse.

You may never be able to alter the size of your joints or the shape of your muscles, but enormous changes are possible through intelligent training and eating programs. The truth of it is we don't all have (and shouldn't want to have) model-perfect bodies, but every one of us can become more fit, more shapely, more toned. If you doubt our words, you'll be converted by the makeover profiles that appear in this chapter.

The payoff to shaping up is that feeling better about your body equals feeling better about yourself, about what you've accomplished on its behalf (Yours is the only body you have, and it gets you through life, so respect it!), and consequently about what you're capable of accomplishing when you put your mind, body, and will to any task.

4. *I'll never look as good as she does.* Nothing destroys motivation faster than seeing somebody else's beautiful, apparently no-maintenance physique. Actually, though, there are few individuals blessed with naturally proportioned, firm, and graceful physiques.

Instead of seizing on these rare figures of perfection as an excuse to do nothing, accept the differences in our species and vow to do your best— for you and only you. As long as you're focused on others, whether in envy or in awe, you'll never get the best results, in your workouts and in your life. You must develop tunnel vision and focus inward, concentrating only on your body and yourself.

5. *I'd like to look and feel better, but it takes so long.* If you're anticipating instant, amazing results from exercise, you're looking for a miracle, not a fitness program. That's as if you've just started in the mailroom of a Fortune 500 corporation and fully expect to become the CEO in a matter of days. The fact is, anything worth having usually requires sustained effort and hyper-focus; fitness is no exception.

As we've said, one of the major pluses of The FIRM workout is that you can see results in ten sessions, but we're not talking about total transformation. We're talking about sufficient positive results to keep you with the program. Stay with it, and over time, you'll be surprised at how much firmer, leaner, and more energetic you have indeed become. Remember, any system that promises instant results is guilty of false merchandising.

6. *I'm hopelessly overweight. Why should I even bother to exercise?* Take a deep breath: It's not hopeless.

Scientifically, there's no question about the single most important component of long-term weight loss—regular exercise. Which method works best? Many people are so weak (from having too little muscle and too much fat) that they can't begin to exercise by doing aerobics.

The FIRM invented the smartest and fastest method with aerobic weight training. As we've said, these workouts give up to *three times the fat loss* of high-impact aerobics. Nothing motivates like fast results! And because weights/aerobics combination training causes less breathlessness than ordinary aerobics, overweight beginners enjoy it more.

Of course, moderate calorie restriction must be part of your fitness plan. Make gradual—not drastic—changes in your diet (you'll learn just how to do this in the next chapter, FIRM FUEL), and continue to get some form of exercise every day. Read The FIRM makeovers for proof positive that there *is* hope for you.

7. *I'm forty-five years old. It's just too late for me!* No way! In fact, it's the perfect time to commit to a workout program.

After your initial two-week break-in period, you will make rapid, dramatic gains for about the first sixty days! By the third week, you will already see visible changes in muscle tone and body shape.

Like younger exercisers, middle-agers are initially motivated by fat loss and improved body shape. But all ages soon realize that half the benefits are mental. As Socrates noted in the fifth century B.C., "Vigorous exercise fills a man with pride and spirit; and he becomes twice the man he was." Obviously, the same goes for women!

After a few weeks of working out, you'll realize you sleep more soundly. You'll gradually feel stronger, more energetic, more optimistic, and less depressed! Depression, by the way, afflicts about 40 percent of older Americans. Research shows that exercise is at least as effective as psychotherapy—but much cheaper and faster. (In 1976, John H. Greist, a professor of psychiatry at the University of Wisconsin, found that running helped people overcome depression, and in a later study at Tufts University, researchers verified that, like aerobic exercise, strength training has a strong antidepressant effect—"virtually all" of the test subjects experienced some relief from depression.)

As an older exerciser, you'll need more time to recover between workouts, better nutrition, and more sleep at night. When you begin, working out every other day will be about right—and keep in mind that you should initially do a little less of the workout than you think you can.

Once you're really in shape, seriously expect to be operating twenty years *below* your chronological age. In other words, a forty-five-year-old exerciser will have the same strength/endurance/energy level as a twenty-five-year-old nonexerciser.

Even in the elderly, weight training has a miraculous ability to reverse aging. In one eight-week study at prestigious Tufts University, women in their nineties actually tripled their strength—with weights! If people understood this amazing scientific research, they'd be saying, "I'm too old *not* to exercise!"

8. *Exercise, yuckkk! Boring, boring, boring!* Hey, let's not generalize here. It's true that much, even most, exercise is boring—as well as frustrating, especially if you can't keep up with the "Aerobics Instructor from Planet Babe." And virtually all video workout tapes are beyond boring—they're stultifying (and often unsafe, as well). Which means, of course, that you use them once, and they're history.

But there are so many exercise options that aren't boring in the least— in-line skating and bike riding, for instance. Tennis, swimming, or pickup basketball can be extremely pleasurable. Even treadmills and stationary bikes, if you bring your Walkman, listen to your favorite music, and meditate—precious time to spend only with yourself! And, best of all, when you're concentrating on any physical activity, the cares of the day get crowded out. That's all anyone can ask for!

However, when Anna devised The FIRM program, she was hyperaware of boredom and did everything to prevent it from creeping into workouts. That's one of the reasons for interval training and cross training: varying the types of exercise so you stay stimulated and alert. It's also the reason that The FIRM classes and videos have leaders and members with whom you can bond. Consider getting a personal trainer at least a few times a week, and/or work out or do a sports activity with a friend or spouse. Exercise bonding is a very real, very positive occurrence, and it lasts!

9. *Nothing, I mean nothing, will make my saddlebags go away!* We beg to differ—whether the problem is saddlebags, a spare tire, protruding belly, or sagging arms or butts. All truly effective programs will change your *total* body.

Saddlebags are simply female-specific fat deposits on the outside of the thighs. For many women these are the last fat deposits to shrink, but shrink they will. The pitted fat comprising saddlebags is called cellulite, but fat is fat, and fat is cellulite. No magic eighty-dollar jar of cream is going to get rid of it. And neither will starving yourself.

The only way to get rid of cellulite is by working those areas with aerobic weight training. When you're burning fat at three times your normal rate, some of it will be the cellulite. While requiring long-term commitment to fitness, saddlebags are removable without liposuction!

10. *Exercise? I just don't feel like it!* Make no mistake about it, your mind can really do a number on your body, tricking it into laziness and sabotaging your fitness goals. It can create any one or several of a million excuses not to exercise. If you're too tired, then exercise for energy. If you're too hungry, then exercise, burn fat, raise your metabolism, and you'll be able to eat more. If you're too full, work it off with exercise. For every lame excuse, there's a practical, scientifically tested rebuttal.

But to avoid letting your mind prevail with these common and empty excuses, you must mentally train to think like a warrior and to focus on a single goal: becoming the best that you can be.

DEAR FIRM

"FIRM workouts are fun, very sound and thorough, and they work! Aerobics and weights cover all aspects of fitness training. And now that I'm approaching menopause, exercise is more important than ever to maintain good health."

SHAWN SHEFFIELD, 40,
homesteader, Pace, Florida

RENEE HOLLER

AGE: 38   PROFESSION: HOMEMAKER

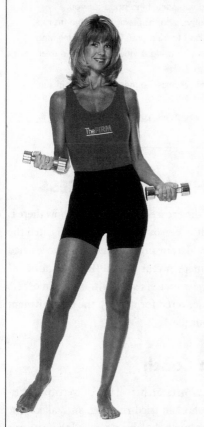

Tall and beautifully conditioned, Renee has been coming to The FIRM for three years and instructing for one.

Renee had always tried to keep in shape, but after giving birth to three children, she'd put on pounds and was having back trouble. Her doctor told her she needed to lose weight and to strengthen her abs and recommended The FIRM workout. The rest is history.

This instructor is very big on instilling fun into the workout. "I think if the instructor is not motivated and not having a good time, it filters into the delivery.

I smile and cut some jokes a couple of times. One of the best compliments clients can pay you is to come up and say that they never looked at the clock and the class is already over!"

Renee feels that many students identify with her because a lot of them are her age, some are more settled than the younger instructors, a lot of them have kids as she does. "I think," she muses, "they like having someone up there like them."

When asked why The FIRM appeals to women like herself, Renee replies, "A lot of different things. What made me join initially was to try to get my weight down and my health improved. Some women do it because it's their release. They come here stressed. They have an hour to themselves to do something totally for themselves. And some long-timers, like me, just love doing it!"

(continued)

RENEE'S TIPS FOR BEGINNERS:

○ When you work out, don't think about your to-do list or your kids.

○ Concentrate only on you and doing something good for you.

○ No matter what type of workout you do, appreciate that the instructor is there to be approached and to help you. If there's something you don't understand, ask. If you're using a video, replay the exercise several times, study it, learn it.

○ Two major pluses to weight maintenance—mineral and vitamin supplements and protein drinks.

○ Have fun with your workout. If you don't, you won't go on doing it.

COMMITMENT—THE KEY TO SUCCESS

All right, we've taken care of all the excuses, and you now know there is no valid reason for a normally healthy person of any age not to catch the fitness bug. Commitment, however, like any other virtue, must be learned until it becomes automatic. For nineteen years, The FIRM has done research to find out what makes some exercisers stick with it, while others quit. Here are the principles we discovered for making the commitment process a quick and firm part of your life.

Get a Coach

Coaching works! As far back as 1976, researchers at the University of Wisconsin studied a group of people who had tried running, and failed. The dropouts were given a coach, and twelve weeks later almost all these people were running successfully. That's why, as we've already said, every FIRM video stars a leader who functions as your personal coach and with whom you bond.

As your personal at-home coach, FIRM instructors bring thousands of hours of actual teaching experience to you. They know the challenges of completing certain exercise sequences, and they perform the workout right along with you. Since most of the cast members are FIRM clients or instructors, you actually have a group of "comrades" who create a team spirit through the workouts.

Remember what we said a few pages ago. Whether it be with a spouse, workout buddy, or personal trainer—establish an emotional/intellectual tie with that person. And if you have young children at home, set aside a special exercise hour every day for *all* of you! It'll keep you going. Even in times when you don't feel like exercising, the commitment to another will propel you forward!

DEAR FIRM

"I know I need weights to prevent osteoporosis. The FIRM lets me go at my own pace and move up or down as needed on a certain day. If I don't exercise, I get sluggish, a little down. I guess I'm hooked!"

PAMELA ROGERS, 42,
marketing consultant, Boulder, Colorado

Have Clear Reasons to Change

Pinpoint that aspect of your body that you'd most like to change. Take a realistic look. Please don't exaggerate your problems. Just be as honest and clear-sighted as possible. Once you rationally and calmly focus on your target, and know there's a solution, you're *motivated!*

Exercisers soon discover that half the benefits of exercise are mental: better sleep, less depression, more creative energy, more joie de vivre.

Positively Visualize Your Outcome

Imagine, as clearly as you can, your new life as an exerciser. Think of the clothes you'll be able to wear. Think of having the strength and energy to enjoy more of life. Think of enlarging your social circle. Think of losing your anxiety about becoming old and weak. Think of yourself as taking control of your life. Basically, of course, you'll be the same person you are now—only significantly healthier and happier! The miracle of exercise is that it works on every level of being, not just the physical!

However, it's important not to get carried away with unrealistic expectations; researchers at the University of Scranton compared people who kept their New Year's fitness resolutions with those who didn't. Those who kept their promises shared these three traits.

1. They believed in their ability to change.
2. They did not indulge in self-blame.
3. They avoided wishful thinking, such as "My life will change completely if I get in shape."

One exerciser told us she was always able to motivate herself by thinking about the comparison we'd once made between a workout and a coat of paint: Working out (especially with weights) very quickly makes you start to feel better, but visible results require more than one workout because results occur on a microscopic level. Think of each workout as a coat of paint—each session adds a layer here and removes a layer there. Imagine how different a chair looks after twenty coats of paint. After forty layers. After one hundred. So it is with workouts.

This paint comparison allowed the exerciser to visualize the eventual reward of her long-term plan. She told us that no matter how tired or rushed she was, she said to herself, "Here goes one more coat of paint," and started her workout.

When exercisers say working out is 90 percent mental, they're right. How well you maintain concentration, intensity, and a positive attitude will decide whether your results are so-so or great. If an overweight exerciser sees working out as "torture for letting myself get fat," she will soon be a dropout.

Each workout is a challenge. You win just by playing. Whatever happens in the rest of the world, your body will always be a bit better than it was yesterday. What could be more positive than that?

DEAR FIRM

"I convinced my parents (both in their mid-fifties) to try The FIRM—plus now they hike, bike, and sea kayak. I'm so proud of them!"

MEGAN WEIR, 28,
front desk clerk for resort, Jackson, New Hampshire

"I feel strong and have great energy. Since using The FIRM, I look much better after having three kids than before kids!"

NICOLE TODD, 36,
homemaker, Bridgewater, New Jersey

Know the Method Will Work

At the beginning of any workout program, it's important you spend time learning. You must become informed about the method you have chosen so that you know with absolute certainty that it will work to accomplish your specific goal. This is exactly what we've tried to help you with in FIRM FACTS (chapter 2).

Gaining basic scientific knowledge is the most important key to motivation. Without a practical knowledge of the processes by which exercise works, it's very difficult to work your way to a great body.

Again and again the public fails at exercise because it lacks knowledge. Here are the two principal knowledge-related reasons people fail:

Reason number one: *Workouts are unbelievably boring unless you know what happens inside a contracting muscle:* what makes it grow or shrink and what makes the fat layer change. When you master the basics, it all becomes fascinating because you know what you're doing. You know how to work with it to make it stronger, leaner, and healthier.

Knowledge also makes you able to work harder and able to make your body change faster. It is impossible, for example, to make abdominal exercises work as well when you don't know where your muscles are and how to feel them. Knowledge makes the difference between faking your way through a set of crunches (no result) and being able to visualize the working muscle, contracting it fully on each set (great results).

Reason number two: *Knowledge lets you evaluate the effectiveness of your workout.* Without a working knowledge of the basics, you can only assume that the designer of your workout did a good job. You can only assume that you will eventually get results. You can only assume you are performing the moves well.

Solid motivation cannot be built on flimsy assumptions. Assumptions make it easy to doubt your course of action. It is impossible to believe in your ability to change if you have doubts about your workout's effectiveness.

Beginners should actually spend more time learning than working out. *FIRM for Life* provides you with just that opportunity—between covers!

"Results, results, results!!! I've seen the change in my leg shape, thighs, buttocks, and upper arm muscles, and I can't imagine quitting The FIRM."

CHRISTINE KEYES, 40,
litigation specialist

Commit to Twenty-One Workouts— Then One Hundred

Behavioral scientists tell us that it takes twenty-one repetitions for a new habit to become established. After one hundred repetitions, the new habit becomes automatic. To start a workout program, you *must* commit to doing it for twenty-one sessions—no matter what. Mark your calendar with specific workout times.

After twenty-one workouts, you'll be seeing and feeling results. Motivated by your initial success, committing to making it through the full one hundred is much easier. Always keep in mind that good habits are as hard to break as bad ones.

Immediate Action Toward the Goal

Once you've learned the scientific workings of your chosen workout program, set goals, made the necessary alterations in your lifestyle and your fuel, and committed to the twenty-one workouts, go for it at once!

At The FIRM, we keep records. We know exactly what the beginner should expect from FIRM workouts: After the initial two-week break in phase, your body will continue to make rapid, dramatic progress for the first sixty days. During your third week, you will be able to see visible improvement in your muscle tone and overall body shape. Then get ready to hurdle the Golden Hundred!

"For once, I can stay with an exercise program!"

MARY BEAL, 26,
recruitment coordinator, Arlington, Virginia

Develop the Exercise Habit

As we age, we realize that exercise is essential to good health *and* good looks. Regular exercise should be as automatic as brushing your teeth or doing laundry. It's ironic that we're taught at an early age to be fastidious about certain aspects of self care, and yet care of the body is almost neglected. We're taught to take better care of our cars! When we view life as a continuous learning experience, learning new self-care that makes us more attractive and more effective can be exciting.

Our grandfather Benson once told us, "We do what we want to do." Having time to exercise, as we mentioned before, is doable when you *determine your priorities*. A major goal of working out, of course, is looking better, but that's only a part of why it should be one of your top priorities.

We've all heard that we don't value our health until we lose it. With today's insurance and health care costs and the specter of old age, we must do what we can to keep ourselves healthy and youthful. All of us have read so many scientific findings about the health benefits of exercise that we take it as a given.

Commit to the exercise habit. Focus on benefits. You can be a younger, shapelier, more energetic, and contented individual for the rest of your life.

Make Exercise a Priority

It all comes down to mindset. Think about results. What will make you look more beautiful in more situations: a three hundred dollar dress, an eight hundred dollar suit, or thirty workouts that tone your overall body?

Just how do you develop gorgeous legs? By buying Manolo Blahnik shoes or by doing intense leg work? We're certainly not casting aspersions on good clothing, but we are saying that it's crucial to your overall well-being that you begin working on a valuable foundation.

Exercise can make you feel more beautiful than a closet full of new clothes can. And when you're in good, firm, lean, graceful shape, you'll flatter the clothes, not vice versa. We've already said that vanity is a great motivator. And what gives a man or a woman more personal pride than a body that's in maximally good shape?

DEAR FIRM

"I had never, ever, ever been able to stick with an exercise program before. With The FIRM, the results are so fast and dramatic and motivating that I can't stop. After three years, I'm still seeing improvement."

**RENEE C., 27,
master control operator for TV station, Kansas City, Missouri**

Increase Physical Activity Throughout the Day

To offset a sedentary lifestyle, you have to insert action into your day every chance you get. We've mentioned America's addiction to TV—hours and hours of doing nothing, frequently combined with eating high-fat, high-sugar junk. Here's the plain, honest truth: Our obsession with television restricts us so much that we're becoming increasingly resistant to real-world activities.

Like any other endeavor you set out to accomplish by yourself—whether it's starting a business or building a great new body—you're going to have to be prepared to make some sacrifices, and sedentary activity is chief among them.

Your new formula goes like this: Always strive to increase your activity level during the day—for instance, walk instead of drive, climb stairs instead of taking the elevator.

Supplement workouts with activities like biking, running (great for the heart, lungs, circulation, and endurance), swimming (great for resistance training), or outdoor sports such as tennis, volleyball, or softball. All kinds of physical activity are good for you, and variety helps keep you motivated to be active.

Demand the Right Kind of Fuel

You'll learn much more about proper nutrition in our FIRM FUEL chapter, but here's a brief explanation of why you are what you eat.

Metabolism is the rate at which your body burns calories. During workouts, you exhaust glycogen, a form of carbohydrate stored in your muscles. With proper nutrition along with exercise, you'll build additional layers of muscle during recovery and increase your metabolic rate. If you're trying to reduce your fat layer, you must refuel the calories burned in exercise sessions with carbohydrates and proteins, avoiding excess sugar and fats.

Even though it's no longer considered advisable to get locked into counting calories, it's important to know what's happening calorically when you exercise. For example, each FIRM workout burns about 250 to 300 calories. Each power walking session burns about 150 to 250 calories. (These estimates vary with the level of intensity, length of workout, and heaviness of the weights.) Any vigorous exercise session of about thirty to forty minutes burns about 200 to 250 calories. But please don't begin obsessing about the synergy of calories and exercise: Eat prudently, exercise regularly, and you'll get the results you desire without driving yourself nuts.

The major point here is that cutting calories alone is never enough; if you want to lose fat, you must increase your activity level. Fuel for exercise is also fuel for your brain. You have to eat smart and break a sweat in order to attain lean good looks.

DEAR FIRM

"The FIRM makes me feel fabulous. Endorphin highs are great!"

DONNA RUNTE, 28,
health care administrative assistant, Milwaukee, Wisconsin

JANET BRUNSON

AGE: 34   PROFESSION: LAWYER

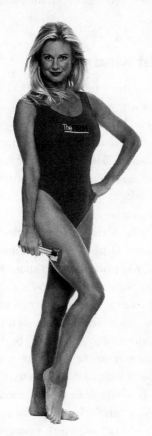

It's difficult to picture gentle, lovely Janet as a fiercely combative trial lawyer, but that's what she was. In fact, she began coming to The FIRM as a client while she was in law school—a heavy schedule to handle. But, as she says, "It was a wonderful release. I was happy. At the time, I didn't realize how much the exercise and being at The FIRM and being part of The FIRM contributed to that."

Once her legal career swung into high gear, Janet, who was working seventy hours a week, didn't have time to devote to exercise; she took a year off and then came back to The FIRM. Next she married and when she got pregnant stopped working out again. After her daughter, Brooks, was born, she ceased practicing law; she loved being a mom, but nevertheless, she needed a challenge. So back she came to The FIRM until she and her husband relocated to Atlanta for two years, where she found no workout routine that could hold a candle to aerobic weight training. When they returned to Columbia, Janet made a beeline for The FIRM and stayed, eventually becoming an instructor. There's something equalizing about The FIRM, which Janet applauds.

"You know," she muses, "our clients are happy. We have clients who are physically gorgeous and we have clients who are slightly

(continued)

overweight but still work out. They're very motivational for us. . . . I've never been overweight but I've been in the position where I wanted something so badly (I wanted to teach) that I know how they feel."

And what about the balanced lifestyle The FIRM recommends? "That's it," Janet agrees. "When I look into the eyes of the instructors, the clients, or people I know, I feel that balance. It makes me feel centered. It makes me feel very human, very real, and very equal. That's where my strength comes from."

JANET'S TIPS FOR BEGINNERS:
○ Make yourself stick it out for ten workouts, when you'll see results.
○ Don't feel ashamed if you're out of shape or overweight.
○ Start making the necessary lifestyle adjustments right away.
○ Read this book and/or don't fast-forward through the informational section at the beginning of the videotapes.
○ Think about what you eat.
○ Think about the alcohol you drink—it's a depressant and makes you physically weaker.
○ Set achievable goals—in workouts and in life.

Learn How to Concentrate During Workouts

A high degree of intensity and focus makes exercise work, so don't let anything distract you. When you work out, your exercise space should become the center of your universe. All of your senses must be directed toward your workout and your workout only. Your breathing, your weights, and your movements rule the space. Of course, focus is also a matter of safety, but above all, it gives you special time to free your mind and body of tension and totally embrace a remarkable sense of well-being. Casual chatter, answering the phone, and other distractions can destroy your concentration and open the door for lower intensity, injury, or quitting.

There really is a certain workout Zen, or inner-directedness. This attitude of acceptance is the hallmark of the mature exerciser: He or she accepts the assignment and its duration, and simply adapts to it. By eliminating the stress of indecision, the job—any job, in exercise or living—becomes much easier.

Over the years, we've developed our own concentration techniques. We narrow our vision and don't let our eyes stray. We focus on alignment and pay attention to how our muscles are interacting with each other. We feel our breath going in and out of our bodies, and we know when our oxygen need is increasing. Focusing is like meditation: It takes practice.

If you are to succeed, you must concentrate solely on your muscles and how they are responding to the stress of exercise. Only then will you be able to maximize your energy and achieve great results.

DEAR FIRM

"My entire body has changed since The FIRM! My arms are shapely, no more hanging flab! I have rippled abs! My legs and calves are awesome and my buttocks are almost rock solid. I have maintained this shape for two and a half years. My husband says he never dreamed I could look this way! We've been married eleven years, and it seems like we just got married again!"

LYNNE G., 29,
child development assistant, Hayward, California

Recover from the Workouts

Rest is an essential component of fitness. Take naps whenever possible and get plenty of sleep. Remember, even when you're sleeping, your muscles are burning fat. We recommend that everyone, but especially those over thirty-five, pay special attention to the recovery process.

Proper stretching, whirlpools, heat treatments, and massage are all ways to assist recovery after exercise. Massage is a wonderful physical and emotional therapy that reduces stress and may speed muscle recovery.

Intense, physical workouts are maximized with special fuels. Many professionals use a variety of simple and complex carbohydrates sixty to ninety minutes prior to a workout. The need for refueling, especially protein, should be met within thirty minutes after workouts to maximize your gain. Don't waste time and energy by not properly replenishing your body!

STEPHANIE CORLEY

AGE: 24
PROFESSION: HIGH SCHOOL ENGLISH TEACHER

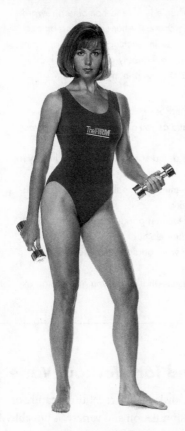

Hearty, healthy, and with commitment oozing out of every pore, Stephanie Corley was clearly born to teach.

Stephanie came to The FIRM through the videos, which she began using religiously her senior year in high school. When she moved from Aiken, South Carolina, to Columbia to attend college, she heard about a gym called The FIRM but didn't realize at first that it was the place the tapes came from. Now, several years later, Stephanie is a FIRM instructor.

She was teaching with The FIRM when she was getting her master's in education, and she feels that, as she says, "it was great training for actual classroom teaching. It was wonderful. It was just coming into a room full of some thirty-odd people and knowing that you're responsible for one hour of a good workout was a lot of pressure. I was so nervous my first class. Scared to death. It really prepared me to face a room full of sixteen-year-old juniors."

Stephanie remembers when her fifty-year-old mother did Jane Fonda, but is proud to report she's now a FIRM Believer. "I remember thinking," Stephanie recalls, "that once you hit twenty-five your body was no longer beautiful, that it was all downhill. Now I realize if you stay healthy, you'll get that beauty that comes from health. I see a lot

(continued)

of high school girls just torturing themselves with this diet and that diet, looking for the magic pill. It absolutely, without doubt, requires physical activity."

Engaged to be married, Stephanie is able to combine a rewarding personal life with two teaching careers. After conducting an exercise class, she claims, "I just feel better. In teaching, you give and give and give all day. I just feel like I cannot honestly give to those kids unless I've taken care of me, and that shows up in my workout."

STEPHANIE'S TIPS FOR BEGINNERS:
○ Start slowly, do what you can, and as you get stronger, increase your intensity.
○ Be inspired by knowing you're doing something that's so hard yet so good for your body.
○ Begin with a strong motivation—mine was health, since there's a history of breast cancer in my family.
○ Admit you love the prospect of looking good—maybe that's vanity, but nobody likes to not fit into their clothes.
○ Craze or fad diets are going to work against your exercise resolve; adopt a healthy eating style.
○ Always strive to challenge yourself—that's how you grow as an exerciser and human being.

Acknowledge the Need for Workout Variety

The best way to stay fit is to acknowledge the repetitious nature of exercise and to give yourself as much stimulation and variety as possible. As we've mentioned, FIRM videos are designed to keep you involved by frequently changing activities and props. There are many mix-and-match possibilities within each video.

With newly acquired muscle strength, you'll be able to participate in sports that were once off limits. Cross training with other activities is made possible by The FIRM's aerobic weight training. You'll have core strength, and an athletic body for everything you do in life. The FIRM prepares you to pick up any weekend sport safely and with confidence.

DEAR FIRM

"The FIRM works. Results don't lie. It's fun to give your real age and watch people just about fall over because they can't believe how old you really are!"

CARLA A. HARLAN, 43,
stockbroker, Clearwater, Florida

Acknowledge the Mental Benefits of Exercise

First motivated by physical changes, exercisers soon feel unexpected physical and emotional perks. University of Wisconsin psychiatry professor Dr. John Greist found, as we've mentioned, that exercise was as effective as psychotherapy in helping people overcome depression.

Exercise alleviates depression for three reasons:

1. People are much happier when their bodies look and feel better.
2. Changing your body empowers you, making you realize that you can change *other* aspects of your life: Look at exercise as an organic antidepressant that you create and control yourself.
3. The rush of endorphins creates a natural euphoria.

One fascinating bit of research found that the euphoric hormonal changes of the exerciser's high are identical to the biochemical changes responsible for the positive feelings experienced by churchgoers after a Sunday service.

Beginners, however, should not expect a postworkout high. In fact, they often feel mentally shot. Why? One study indicated that the exerciser's high often takes several weeks to kick in—after body chemistry adjusts to the new demands of working out.

Add Exercise to Your Emotional Center

The emotional center is that place from which you relate to your dearest concerns: spouse, family, work, friends, spiritual values, and even money (how popular it is to disparage that idea nowadays). Critical to good health, exercise makes you more effective in realizing *all* the things you value most. Laziness, overeating, and overdrinking are all part of life, but when they are a focus of your emotional center, other things suffer. Health and the higher, timeless, universal values cannot flourish. Incorporate exercise into your emotional center, and life's greatest treasures are suddenly within your grasp.

A *Psychology Today* poll indicated that feeling superior to sedentary types is a major source of exercisers' motivation. So get motivated and enjoy a justified moment of superiority. Ninety-three percent of Americans claim fitness is very important to leading a full life, yet only about 10 percent work out regularly and vigorously.

Look at it this way: Getting in shape isn't easy, but living life out of shape is very, very hard!

DEAR FIRM

"Thanks to The FIRM, I believe I will be healthier in my fifties and sixties than I was in my thirties. My energy level is the best it has been in ten years."

THERESA VERNON, 39,
acupuncturist/herbalist

Toughness Training

The urge to improve ourselves is a manifestation of the best in human nature. But the path is exacting. Since goals test you on a profound level, many people never display the spirit to master the steps to personal fulfillment. You must have courage if you want to realize your unique gifts. Many people begin this journey with fitness goals; they're easier to monitor, and you will be able to see your results!

The benefits of a regular diet or fitness program are psychological as well as physical. When people discover they have the tenacity to follow a course of self-improvement, they immediately experience a surge in self-confidence. And as they begin to feel better about themselves, they want to repeat the experience. Even small improvements in eating or exercise habits create the desire to duplicate the success. The same skills that improve physical habits can be applied to other, more abstract, dimensions of life. As we practice new habits, we build confidence in self-mastery through repetition. Paradoxically, this creates the freedom to try new things.

Inner toughness is an acquired skill, and it can be learned. Take a look at these essential, progressive steps for personal change. Since each one builds upon the previous one, don't expect immediate results. Respect the slow nature of change. Don't be afraid to acknowledge the difficulty of the necessary hard work and practice. Know you are on the only worthwhile path to personal fulfillment. If you want to be everything you can be, you must commit to practicing toughness skills.

Jim Loehr in his landmark work, *Toughness Training for Sports: Achieving Athletic Excellence* (Lexington, Mass.: The Stephen Greene Press, 1982), came up with the following ingredients that are imperative if you want to reach your fitness goal, or any other goal in life, for that matter.

- **Self-Discipline**   Any wild force of nature is improved by pruning. You can start this process on the most tangible level, your body! Gain control over the physical dimension by committing to regular systematic training. Begin the groundwork for truly worthwhile accomplishments as you decide to forego short-term pleasures.
- **Self-Control**   As you begin to apply self-discipline in your daily schedule, you will experience self-control. New habits will develop and make it easier to regulate your lifestyle. You will begin to control your food intake, adhere to a workout schedule, and exercise restraint over unhealthy habits.
- **Self-Confidence**   Daily practice of self-control builds a new foundation of behaviors. New habits with visible, measurable outcomes will allow you to trust and rely upon yourself. You will feel assured that you will perform in a predictable, positive manner.
- **Self-Realization**   One day, new accomplishments will announce the birth of a different, more highly crafted person with a deep core of inner strength. This is the magnificent result of toughness training. Throughout a lifelong journey, these four steps make it possible to fulfill the ultimate goal: to be the best that you can be!

FIRM **SUCCESS STORY**
JOANNE JANICKI

"The weights made all the difference. . . ."

I started out as an overweight child and entered adulthood overweight. When I graduated from the University of Florida, I was 5'6" and weighed 216 pounds. The thought of going to job interviews in the corporate world petrified me because I hated the way I looked in a business suit (or anything else, for that matter).

I began a very sensible diet of fruit and vegetables with low-fat protein sources. I also eliminated junk food. The first few weeks were very difficult, but by the fourth week, I felt much better and had much more energy. I didn't miss my high-fat, high-sugar diet.

I began to purchase fitness and weight-loss magazines that published success stories of other women who had lost weight through diet and exercise. These stories motivated me to get physically active. I started out walking and began to see great results both on the scale and in the way I felt. Once the hot Florida summer rolled around, I decided to try an exercise video. My concentration was on aerobics since it was the most touted method for weight loss at the time. Then I hit a dreaded plateau that lasted nearly a year. By that time, I had lost about fifty pounds over the course of a couple of years. I increased the frequency and duration of my aerobics-only workouts with minimal to no results.

I saw a detailed ad for The FIRM videos in one of my magazines and decided to give it a try since I had never incorporated weights into my

(continued)

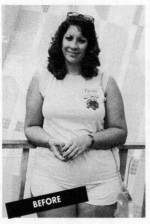
BEFORE

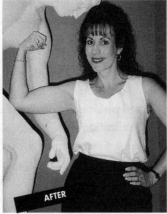
AFTER

workout program. That was about three and a half years ago, and I haven't looked back since, nor have I used any of my other workout videos again! I lost twenty-one more pounds and was afforded more freedom in my food plan since my new muscles helped me burn so many more calories! I could not believe how quickly I saw results. The weights made all the difference in the world! Here are some of my personal tips for success:

- Keep a food diary and write down everything you eat, even if you have a bad food day.

- Try to work out at least five times per week. On the days when you really don't feel like it, start anyway. If you still don't want to continue fifteen minutes into the workout, take a day off. (Chances are you'll keep going!)

- If you slip in your exercise or eating plans, don't beat yourself up—just start out fresh the very next day. Don't wait for another Monday to roll around.

- Take lots of photos on your road to fitness—the results will keep you motivated.

—Joanne Janicki, 32, claims adjuster, Tampa, Florida

FIRM **SUCCESS STORY**
LAURA BAHRENBURG

"It's really true: In just ten workouts, you do see the difference!"

A little over a year ago, I embarked on one of the biggest commitments I have ever made. I had come to the realization that I was thirty-four years old and that time was running out. I weighed 240 pounds, and unless I made a change soon, I would spend the rest of my life over-weight. I modified my diet and designed an exercise program that I could live with. One hundred pounds later, I am a FIRM Believer!

My day starts at 5:30 every morning with one of your workouts. My friend and I rotate Body Sculpting Basics, Low-Impact Aerobics, and Aerobic Interval Training. Your tapes have helped me look the way I do today. I've tried a variety of other exercise programs and none of them targets as many problem areas with the speedy results of The FIRM. It's really true: In just ten workouts, you do see the difference! These results encourage me to go on—I look forward to my workouts because I know I am getting the results promised. I cannot thank your company enough for helping me sculpt the body I've always dreamed of having.

—Laura A. Bahrenburg, 36, homemaker, Carol Stream, Illinois

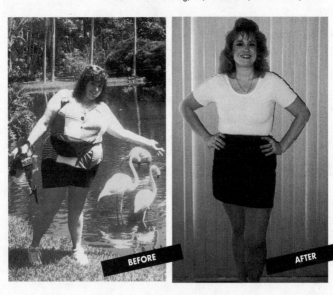

BEFORE

AFTER

FIRM **SUCCESS STORY**
CHARLOTTE LINDLER

"My new nickname is 'Slenderella'!"

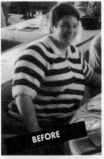

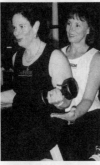

BEFORE

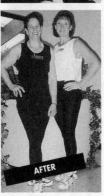

AFTER

Having practiced medicine for eighteen years, I knew better than anyone that I had to lose weight—but nothing worked. Not walking. Not dieting. Being a doctor made things worse—I was supposed to know how to eat correctly! But I just could not stay on a diet.

My motivation and eventual success came from a resolution to lose weight for my twentieth medical school reunion. I found a wonderful personal trainer at The FIRM in Debbie Boyer; she's been the secret of my success. In February of 1996, I was a size twenty-two. I began training with Debbie three, then five times a week. I stopped watching TV because I was in the habit of eating while I watched. I began to add more physical activity whenever possible, like taking stairs instead of the elevator. I also kept a food diary and added more lean animal protein to my diet. My goal was to be physically active for ten hours a week. Debbie even asked me to do quick, eight-minute sessions of abdominal training at night, just like the five-day abs video. After eleven months, I've now lost sixty-seven pounds, and my new nickname is "Slenderella"! My social life is more fun. I have much more energy, I'm happier than ever, and I feel twenty years younger!

I think that one of the most important steps for people trying to lose weight is identifying their motivation. In my case, the reunion was the "hot button" that got me started. Each person has to find their own key to their lock—their own trigger. We're all wired differently, and respond to small but significant new ways of seeing things.

Here are my suggestions for those who want to lose weight, but feel that they just can't:

(continued)

- Change your environment. Avoid the TV—especially if you like to eat while you watch.
- Start slowly. Don't expect everything to happen overnight. Initially, don't over-exert yourself. Set small, achievable goals.
- Results you can see increase your motivation. That's why strength training with weights is perfect.
- Identify your motivational trigger. You've got to find the way to jumpstart your workout program. Once you get started, devote yourself to cultivating your new exercise habit.

—Dr. Charlotte Lindler, 45, pediatrician, Columbia, South Carolina

FIRM **SUCCESS STORY**
ANGIE MARAN

"No one takes me for seventy-two years old. . . ."

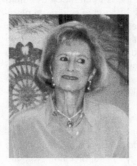

I have been doing The FIRM workouts for more than five years. If it were possible, I would get on a soapbox and travel the country telling senior citizens how positive their attitudes would be if they used The FIRM. There are a lot of exercise tapes on the market, but The FIRM tapes show results much sooner and are very enjoyable to do. I don't get bored. I am addicted! To get people my age motivated, here are some of the phenomenal benefits:

- Excellent for arthritis: I do not have an arthritic joint in my body.
- Circulation: The days I do not exercise, I don't function as well mentally.
- Anti-aging: The blood and moisture to the face lessens wrinkles. Exercise can also reverse muscle and bone loss.
- Balance and coordination: Very helpful—much less risk of broken bones.
- Cosmetic reasons: No one takes me for seventy-two years old. I look fifty-five. My body is trim and toned. My thighs and glutes are as firm as a twenty-five-year-old's.

—Angie Maran, 72, retired, Oak Brook, Illinois

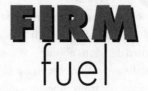

CHAPTER 4

FIRM
fuel

BASIC FACT: If you live on junk food, if you don't get enough sleep, if you don't take care of yourself, you won't have the energy to work out or think clearly. So what we're talking about in *FIRM for Life* is a whole lifestyle, emphasizing diet and nutrition. You really have to look at the whole picture if you want to realize the optimal benefits.

Anna has a friend whose child is in early adolescence (such a fragile time) and whom the mother has put in an exercise class. But when the girl finishes, her mother lets her eat junk food. How can they understand one part of the program and not the other? How can they not know that refueling is as important as reducing? Make no mistake; superior fuel is essential for superior results.

FUELING UP

Visualize yourself as the proud possessor of a body and mind so in tune with life that mere daily activities become filled with genuine joys. It can happen! When physical health and the toning of muscles go hand in hand, you really will attain an enhanced state of well-being you may never have thought possible.

FIRM workouts, as we know, strengthen the heart, lower blood pressure, and trim and sculpt the body to a high level of satisfaction. What a delight to move with ease and grace while doing the most mundane chores!

What personal pride to slip into an old pair of jeans you haven't been able to zip up in years or a slinky Lycra dress.

But to totally get with the program you need to make wise choices about another controllable factor in your life: FIRM Believers strive to make intelligent, informed decisions about their food—the fuel that builds our physical and mental foundation. You have to believe that you get a more rarefied quality of energy from superior foods.

In this chapter we'll describe, in depth, FIRM Fuel, the high nutrient-dense eating plan our clients in the studios and at home have found effective, nonboring, and delicious. Briefly, though, FIRM Fuel is a carefully culled selection of lean meats, green and yellow vegetables, fresh fruits, whole grains, skim milk, and moderate servings of Parmesan cheese, eggs, and fresh nuts.

There is no room in a FIRM Believer's lifestyle for low-end, no-bang, empty-calorie foods that contain little or no vitamins, minerals, amino acids, or essential fatty acids. Your goal is to be well nourished with a high lean-to-fat body composition. By eating well, you'll find it easy to maintain both health and beauty.

For those times when you don't get enough of the right fuel, research has shown that food and vitamin supplements can be helpful. Our first concern, however, is to get you to eat healthfully—and *happily!* Supplements can never fully replace a wisely chosen diet, but they can boost our immune system, fight infections, and generally increase physical and mental performance. Nutritional supplements and food supplements are taken by most athletes.

DEAR FIRM

"Because of The FIRM, I feel great about myself, my clothes fit better, and I am more confident sexually. I don't have to starve myself to lose weight!"

LAURIE M., 29,
psychologist, Florissant, Missouri

FOR WOMEN ONLY

Throughout the ages, in many cultures, mankind has both adored and persecuted women. Some observers of the cult of excessive thinness believe that this fad is just another manifestation of age-old prejudice, and some think it is a desire to "keep women in their place."

Old symptoms of this desire to control women are recorded in history books, and many are not so obvious and are far more subtle. For instance, for many years, American women were denied the right to vote and to hold political office. In early America, a married woman could not totally own and control her own property. When a woman married, her possessions were held in jeopardy of her husband's debts. One of our first South Carolina female ancestors, Mary Stanley, lost all of her money when she had to pay her third husband's gambling debts.

Other cultures also have demeaned women. The Chinese upper class resorted to the torturous practice of binding a female's feet with the tightest of linen strips when the girl was no more than a small child. The result? In adulthood the woman was a virtual invalid and had to be carried by servants throughout her life. Some African cultures put girls in cages at the first sign of menses. Other tribes practice female circumcision.

But not too far behind such horrible practices is the current cult of female thinness we have today. Women (and the society that encourages such deviant behavior) mutilate not just one part of the body, but put strain on and torture all organs by denial of proper food and gross restriction of adequate food. Nature designed the human body for a certain amount of calories each day; it is generally accepted that unless the body receives a minimum of 1,200 calories, the minimum daily recommended amounts (MDR) of building blocks (proteins, carbohydrates, essential fatty acids, vitamins, and minerals) will not be present in the food we eat. Diets that contain too few calories or too few vitamin-mineral rich foods or too many calories from alcohol or "junk foods" cause great harm, especially to the brain, causing symptoms like irritability, lethargy, confusion, temper tantrums, and depression.

We need to know that in order to be beautiful and have abundant energy, we need to build health before we need to think about thinness. Eyes that sparkle, a complexion smooth and silky, hair that looks and feels healthy—how is all this to be achieved?

In addition to exercise, we need to think about food selection. Each food on the pyramid offers important nourishment, and each is important in its own way. Nature designed a marvelous food system for the benefit of mankind. It is up to us to use that food system wisely!

There can be no health on poor diet. Concerning important items, fresh and raw foods would be at the top of our list. We all know people who seem to live on only canned, cooked, processed, dead foods. For them, there never will be a radiant sense of well-being.

NATURE HAS GIVEN EVERYONE A BIRTHRIGHT TO BE BEAUTIFUL

On a recent trip to Jamaica, we were surrounded by a native people of unmistakable beauty and health. In spite of our health education and all of the books we have read on the subject, nothing made an impact on us like this experience. It was the first time we saw physical proof of what our mother had been saying to us for all of these years.

The natural beauty of the Jamaicans was no accident. Time after time, we asked men and women with beautiful faces, teeth, and bodies what they ate when they were growing up. Uniformly, they professed to be poor country people who bought only flour, sugar, and coffee from the local grocers. They grew their meat. They had a cow or goats for milk. Sometimes they boiled the milk, but mostly they drank it fresh and raw. They ate fish, avocados, mangos, and other native vegetables. One girl told us she never had a "hamburger" until she was twenty years old. She said "our poverty protected our health; we were too poor to buy potato chips and cookies." None of these people was overweight. We saw a slender, middle-aged woman eat an entire avocado for lunch. Ironically, most fat-phobic women we know won't touch them. These people proved to us that men and women who are nourished on superior diets of natural unrefined foods are uniformly well formed and healthy.

The media also sanctions a type of peer pressure to eat like everyone else. It is difficult to hold steadfast to a vision of nutritional elitism. To many women, overwhelmed by working and running a household, packaged food seems cheaper and easier to prepare. Manufacturers who spend enormous budgets on advertising are not going to encourage us to learn to seek or use less expensive, more nutrient-rich, natural foods.

We must remember that a diet of packaged, refined foods makes a profound difference in the way children develop and in the way a population looks. Most of us can't see the low level of health in ourselves and our children because of the influence of media. Personalities in television and movies and superstar athletes define who we are. Even though most of us don't look like these rarified examples of beauty, commercial role models continue to exemplify who we think we are.

As a consequence of this deception, we accept inferior nutritional and health standards for ourselves and conceal our failure with expensive cosmetics, dentistry, and cosmetic surgery. We are surrounded by adults in poor health, an epidemic of obesity, and poorly developed children. This is not our destiny! In a country where people eat (ironically, out of poverty!) fresh meats, fruits, and vegetables, they are rich in health and beauty. We all have a choice. Once the damage is done, all the money in the world can't buy what ignorance and greed have robbed from us.

MEET YOUR METABOLISM

Whether or not a major component of your exercise goal is weight loss, you need to understand the nature and function of metabolism.

Metabolism, simply, is the rate at which your body changes food into living tissue and changes living tissue into waste products and energy. No one disputes that there are two basic genetically determined metabolic types, "slow fuel burners" and "fast fuel burners." Slow fuel burners tend to have trouble losing weight, i.e., burning fat; fast fuel burners often have trouble keeping weight on—until the onset of middle-age, when, as we've discussed, the metabolism naturally slows down.

To increase metabolism, you've got to understand two primary concepts: (1) how diet affects metabolism, and (2) how lean body mass, or muscle, is essential to speedier and more efficient fuel-burning.

DEAR FIRM

"I've lost fifty pounds and at thirty-seven years old, I'm in the best shape of my life. The quick and obvious results I got from The FIRM one year ago helped me stick with it. My thighs have the great curves that FIRM instructors' have."

LINDA PASSARETTI, 37,
insurance company employee, Scottsdale, Arizona

DIET AND METABOLISM:
UPGRADING YOUR FUEL

The path to better health is not about an on-and-off diet. Instead, you need to learn new habits to fuel your body for maximal health and well-being, and to adapt to the needs of your internal engine. Build your health; don't strive to become unreasonably thin. Want to know the definition of a good diet? It's *eating for maximum health and performance.*

It is now a scientific given that maintaining a lean, strong body contributes to longevity—so don't think of this new way of eating as a negative state of deprivation. On the contrary, FIRM Fuel is a way of eating the right foods in order to achieve maximal health and performance. Select food for high-quality performance of your internal engine.

Look at it this way: Let's imagine that your body is a car that you need to fuel regularly to make sure it runs. Crucial to it running at peak efficiency is the type of fuel you use. Instead of high-grade gasoline, you might save time and money by adding low-grade kerosene. The car may continue to run, after a fashion, but down the line, you might find that it needs substantial repairs. Gasoline is more expensive, but in the long run, your car "metabolizes" it more efficiently, runs smoother, requires less maintenance, and lasts longer.

You can't cheat your body. You need to eat the right foods in order to boost your metabolism, lose weight, and achieve maximal health and performance. The key to weight loss is consuming fewer empty calories, or low-grade fuel, and increasing caloric expenditure through exercise. To ensure adequate nutrition and the eating of fewer empty calories, we concentrate on a variety of fruits, vegetables, and lean protein while eliminating foods high in fat, sugar, and dangerous chemicals.

DEAR FIRM

"My biggest accomplishment has been keeping off the thirty pounds I lost for three years. I've gone from a size twelve to a size six. I'm also very proud of the muscle definition I have in my arms and legs."

LIZ KARPEL, 31,
director of marketing, St. Louis, Missouri

MUSCLE: THE EFFICIENT FAT BURNER

As we learned in chapter 2, fat is the chief source of energy for your muscles. At rest, muscles burn 70 percent fat, 30 percent sugar. Fat supplies much more "bam" than carbohydrates, and the body has a lot more of it available, almost twice as much. When you're seeking to lose weight through both a healthy diet and regular exercise, and you're not loading your body with fatty foods, your muscles (the most active tissues in your body) will draw from your own accumulated adipose (fat) tissue to keep the motor running.

Because your muscles are always metabolically active, they burn excess body fat—even when you're sleeping. Since the amount of energy produced by the body determines your metabolic rate, the longer and steadier your muscles burn fat, the higher your metabolic rate will become.

That said, we still have to have fuel, and top quality fuel at that. And, although they're not the whole picture, where weight loss is concerned, calories *do* count.

DEAR FIRM

"After retiring from a career in dance, the FIRM has kept me strong and fit. I have strengths now that I never had before. It was a relief to discover that 'retired' doesn't mean overweight and out of shape!"

JULIE PETERSON, 37,
software support worker, Bridgewater, Connecticut

HOW MANY CALORIES
DOES YOUR BODY NEED?

If you are serious about losing weight, start by subtracting 250 calories from your daily caloric intake and incorporate exercise that will burn off 250 more calories (for example, lifting weights for thirty-five minutes or forty-five minutes of brisk walking). This will promote about one pound of fat loss per week. For two pounds of fat loss per week, subtract 750 calories from your daily caloric intake and incorporate exercise that will burn off 250 more. YOU CANNOT LOSE MORE THAN TWO POUNDS OF FAT A WEEK. When you do, you're mainly losing water, which means you're dehydrated, not thinner. And past the two-pound limit, you're also going to be losing muscle mass.

If you would like to gain weight, add 500 to 1,000 calories in order to gain one to three pounds a month.

For permanent results, many experts recommend a weight loss of no more than half a pound a week. While this may seem slow, it prevents your body from returning to its original level, which is programmed through hormonal messengers. Avoid this famine response and take fat off slowly without losing precious muscles.

Our primitive Neolithic ancestors did a great deal of physical work and ate about 2,900 calories a day. Today, most women require about 1,800 calories a day and men about 2,300. An acceptable range for dieting women is 1,300–1,699 a day. But to minimize the body's powerful starvation response, which we discussed in chapter 2, you must make your diet as gentle and invisible as possible: Never miss a meal. Lift weights to maintain precious muscle tissue. And *never ever* go below 1,200 calories a day.

An intake of less than 1,200 calories causes side effects such as irritability, nervousness, and depression. Appropriate dieting should be visualized as less food (one large portion) and more exercise (one additional hour of *vigorous* activity). Do not remove more than one portion of food from a single meal, and never slight breakfast!

WHAT'S WRONG WITH THIS PYRAMID?

Although calories ultimately determine weight loss or gain, the nutrient value of foods can greatly influence your long-term health and how you feel on a daily basis. Sensitive to this, the U.S. Department of Agriculture, Human Nutrition Information Service, and Food Marketing Institute have developed a Food Guide Pyramid, listing the typical adult American's daily nutritional needs.

The USDA pyramid on page 95 is a graphic outline of the three basic sections of your daily nutritional intake of approximately 55 percent car-

JENNIFER CARMEN

AGE: 24   PROFESSION: TECHNICAL RECRUITER

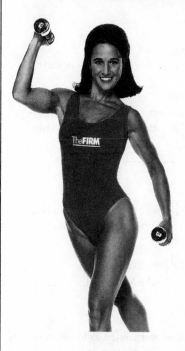

A diminutive, dark-haired woman, Jennifer virtually sparkles—as does her diamond engagement ring—with energy and confidence.

Jennifer initially heard about The FIRM from a friend, and she became a client in order to lose the fifteen pounds she'd gained in college.

"I could not take it off," she recalls. "I tried to do it myself, just running and doing the athletic things I used to do. But I'd kept it on for two and a half years. As you know, it's hard to take off."

After working out with The FIRM for a year, the fifteen pounds were history. Another year later, she's not only back to where she was before she gained the fifteen pounds, but she has also gained muscle. "As far as my clothing size is concerned," she adds, "it's as small as it's ever been."

Jennifer loves teaching *and* working out. Coming to The FIRM is her favorite time of day. "I mean," she says enthusiastically, "I can't wait to get here!"

When asked if she's changed since she joined The FIRM, Jennifer cites accomplishing the goal of getting her weight down and becoming responsible enough to work in the business world for two and a half years.

"I've grown up a lot. I do have a full-time job, and I teach and train, so I really have to be organized," Jennifer says, then adds, "And I have a better understanding of beginners and people losing weight because I've been there. I can truly say this works because I've been there and done that!"

(continued)

JENNIFER'S TIPS FOR BEGINNERS:
- Start off slow.
- Don't expect something to happen overnight.
- Take it on a day-to-day basis.
- Really pay attention to form.
- Make sure you're doing everything correctly.
- Listen to what the instructor is saying—don't try to jump in and do your own thing.
- Be patient and accepting of yourself.
- Maintain a lifestyle based on moderation.
- Keep motivated by telling yourself that strong women are beautiful—inside and out!

bohydrates, 15 percent protein, and 30 percent fat. While analyzing these numbers, remember:

1. Protein, both dairy and meat, can be high in fat.
2. Starchy carbohydrates can be refined, which means they may contain extra sugar or fat.

The basis of the USDA pyramid, at a recommended six to eleven servings, consists of starchy complex carbohydrates including breads, cereals, rice, and pasta—the easiest group for most people to consume. The next largest group (which most of us don't eat enough of) is the vegetable group: The number of recommended daily servings of these fibrous complex carbohydrates is three to five servings. We are told we should consume two to four servings daily of the third largest food group, fruit. Protein is the fourth largest group: The USDA recommends two to three four-ounce servings of dairy products and two to three servings of meat, poultry, fish, dry beans, and nuts. The last and smallest section is fats, which has no recommended serving amount.

So what's the problem with this 55/15/30 percent ratio? According to recent research (*Optimum Sports Nutrition* by Dr. Michael Colgan), the USDA Food Guide Pyramid appears to be based solely on the needs of *sedentary* individuals!

USDA FOOD PYRAMID

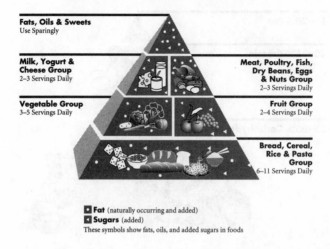

Fats, Oils & Sweets
Use Sparingly

Milk, Yogurt & Cheese Group
2–3 Servings Daily

Meat, Poultry, Fish, Dry Beans, Eggs & Nuts Group
2–3 Servings Daily

Vegetable Group
3–5 Servings Daily

Fruit Group
2–4 Servings Daily

Bread, Cereal, Rice & Pasta Group
6–11 Servings Daily

■ **Fat** (naturally occurring and added)
◀ **Sugars** (added)
These symbols show fats, oils, and added sugars in foods

At The FIRM, we believe that if you wish to live an active life that includes a better figure, a higher level of fitness, enhanced mental acuity, and increased self-esteem, you must understand the importance of quality body fuel in a whole new way. For this reason, we have developed the FIRM Fuel Pyramid.

THE FIRM FUEL PYRAMID

Designed for maximal health and fitness benefits, The FIRM Fuel Pyramid differs from the USDA listing in four primary ways:

1. The percentages of protein and carbohydrates are higher, and fat is lower—*55–65 percent carbohydrates, 20–25 percent protein, 15–20 percent fat* as compared to USDA's 55/15/30 percent.
2. Carbohydrates are not refined and are as close as possible to their pure, natural state (as grown by Mother Nature). They are also divided into two subcategories: *fibrous* and *starchy.*
3. The protein category doesn't contain nuts and beans—but is based completely on low-fat animal protein. If you are a vegetarian, you must

THE FIRM FOOD PYRAMID

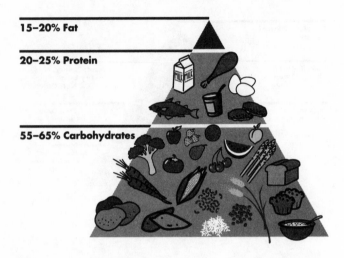

15–20% Fat

20–25% Protein

55–65% Carbohydrates

consume enough nuts and beans to equal the meat source caloric requirements.

4. The fat category is limited to 15–20 percent of total caloric intake and includes only fresh oils with a minimum of saturated fat.

Now let's examine each FIRM Fuel group in more detail.

55–65 PERCENT CARBOHYDRATES— THE ENERGY SOURCE

Carbohydrates fuel the mind and body and should be eaten at regular intervals throughout the day. Natural carbohydrates such as beans, brown rice, and whole fruit enter the bloodstream at a leisurely pace. Because these natural foods supply the preferred time-release energy that lasts for hours, they qualify as *complex* carbohydrates (along with starches). As foods are processed, however, they tend to degrade into less desirable *simple* carbohydrates (sugars). When the fiber is removed from whole grains, the resulting white rice and white flour are classified as simple carbohydrates because they are metabolized much faster—like sugars. When the fiber is removed from whole fruit, the resulting fruit juice is classified as a simple carbohydrate—a sugar. Eating sugary foods puts you on the fast track to obesity, because sugar quickly overloads your bloodstream, which the body strains to normalize by storing the excess sugar as fat. And become sugar calories are metabolized quickly, your hunger soon returns.

For a great workout, eat a portion of *complex* carbohydrates thirty minutes before your workout. (Fruit *juice* is too "simple" and will not do the job.) After working out, eat another serving of complex carbs, accompanied by a serving of protein to help rebuild muscle tissue (since muscle tissue is made of protein). Overall, carbohydrates should make up 55–65 percent of our daily calories, or about 1,100–1,300 of a 2,000-calorie day.

Unrefined Complex Carbohydrates

The most nutritious complex carbohydrates are unrefined and in their natural state; they include grains, legumes, nuts, seeds, and vegetables. Whole fruit is also considered a complex carbohydrate, although it contains sugar in the form of glucose or fructose. Nuts and seeds, although they're formally classified as carbohydrates, contain high amounts of fat and should be eaten in smaller amounts.

Fiber Power

Now on to the two subcategories of unrefined complex carbohydrates, *starchy* and *fibrous*. Most of us eat plenty of starchy carbohydrates, such as pasta and rice, and neglect the fibrous variety, such as asparagus and eggplant.

Those fibrous carbs, frequently green in color, will help you "lean-down" much faster than the starchy ones and are supervaluable as part of a weight loss program. A good daily FIRM Fuel weight loss menu would include starchy carbs—oatmeal or a corn muffin—for breakfast; for lunch, a mix of fibrous and starchy—for instance, lentil soup and a spinach salad; and for dinner, another carb mixture like pasta with steamed vegetables.

Fiber is a crucial part of our fuel, not only because it aids digestion, but also because it controls the rapidity with which carbohydrates enter our bloodstreams: When excess starchy or refined carbs race

FIBROUS AND STARCHY CARBOHYDRATES

FIBROUS	STARCHY
Asparagus	Barley
Green beans	Lima beans
Broccoli	Red beans
Brussels sprouts	Black–eyed peas
Cabbage	Corn
Carrots	Whole-meal flour
Cauliflower	Lentils
Celery	Oatmeal
Cucumbers	Pasta
Eggplant	Peas
Lettuce	Popcorn
Mushrooms	Potatoes
Green peppers	Rice
Red peppers	Sweet potatoes
Spinach	Tomatoes
Squash	Shredded wheat
Zucchini	Yams

Source: *Optimum Sports Nutrition*, by Dr. Michael Colgan

through our systems, the body stores them as fat. Even the sedentary USDA chart advises us to increase fiber's role in our diet by eating:

1. Three to five daily servings of fibrous vegetables: green and red leaves, roots, stems, and nonsweet fruit like tomatoes and yellow peppers
2. Two to four daily servings of fresh, unpeeled fruit
3. Three to five daily servings of such starchy carbs as white and sweet potatoes, corn, beets, brown rice, and other fresh unrefined whole grains

Alternatively, remember that fiber is contained in all unrefined natural state carbs. If you consume unrefined starchy carbs and the USDA recommended five to nine servings of fruits and vegetables, you'll automatically be getting adequate fiber.

To ensure that you're getting the best starchy carbs in grain, upgrade your sources. Search for fresh breads made locally without preservatives.

There is, of course, more to nutrition than just eating the right balance of carbohydrate, fat, and protein. Foods also contain essential trace minerals, fiber, vitamins, and living enzymes. Produced by living cells, enzymes are complex, protein-based substances needed to catalyze, or promote, specific biochemical reactions of metabolism and digestion. Cooking not only reduces a food's usable vitamin, mineral, and fiber content but the cooking temperature utterly destroys all enzymes.

Human biochemistry is so complex that precise cause and effect relationships are extremely difficult to establish. (In *Enzyme Nutrition* by Dr. Edward Howell, it was reported that one authority found ninety-eight distinct enzymes at work in the arteries alone!) But scientists are keenly aware that modern food processing and cooking (both of which remove nutrients) are somehow related to the modern plagues of cancer and degenerative diseases such as arthritis.

It is important to clarify that cooking and food processing are not really the problem. The real problem is America's predominantly all-cooked/all-processed diet. When natural, raw, fresh, enzyme-rich, vitamin-rich foods are diminished until they become just a small percentage of your daily diet, you are in deep trouble. That's why many nutritionists recommend that one third (some say half!) of your daily calories come from raw food like fruit, vegetables, and dark green salads.

Like exercise, the science of nutrition is young and in flux. Much more will be learned in the next forty years, but since we have to eat in the meantime, we must constantly update our information. It's also a smart move to stay a step ahead of the "official" recommendations, because research results are necessarily very slow. No one has forty years to wait around!

Twenty years ago, the medical establishment was still poohpoohing vitamins. Today, the same people profess that vitamins not only promote better health, they can save lives. Likewise, many ideas that are now being dismissed as nonsense by the medical establishment will eventually be proven to have great value. And often an overpriced new prescription will receive more attention than a cheaper herbal cure that is just as effective. For these reasons, it's smart to acquaint yourself with the material in the "alternative" nutrition section of your health food store's reading rack.

Stay away from canned and refrigerated fruit juices—they supply the body with one big dose of simple sugar and no fiber. Choose instead fresh, raw vegetables and fruit juices made with a juicer; when consumed immediately, these are excellent sources of carbohydrates, minerals, and vitamins plus precious enzymes. Fresh fruits and vegetables also contain generous amounts of vitamin C, which increases energy level and simply makes you feel better.

If you're worried about your body's fat level, fuels like these will prove invaluable since they reduce hunger significantly more than do empty carbs—thus the name!

Refined Carbohydrates

Less nutritious carbohydrates include processed food such as white bread, store-bought crackers and cookies, and foods made from refined flour. Avoid packaged and premixed foods whenever possible because of the paucity of their nutrients.

Adjusting your diet will require rethinking menus. The good news is that the healthy foods comprising FIRM Fuel usually require minimal preparation.

DEAR FIRM

"When I started with The FIRM, I weighed 250 pounds, my hips were forty-two inches, my thighs were twenty-four inches, my waist was thirty inches, and my arms twelve inches. A year later—hips thirty-four inches, thighs eighteen and a half inches, waist twenty-two inches, arms ten inches. I wear a size six, and my muscles look great. I have confidence, I look good, I feel good, people mistake me for a twenty-four-year-old. I've had eight children, and no one would ever guess!"

REYLAIN B., 38,
Livingstone, Montana

20–30 PERCENT PROTEIN— BUILDING LEAN BODY MASS

This is the single most neglected, misunderstood aspect of an exerciser's diet. Protein deficiency is without question *the biggest* nutritional reason for lack of progress among the diet-conscious at our studios.* If you're like most people, you may think of protein as being fattening because it is often *accompanied* by fat. The trick is to separate the fat

---

*Be aware that the liver and kidneys can be damaged by extreme, *long-term overdose* of protein. (It breaks down into a toxic ammonia called urea.) By helping the body to flush out urea, drinking a generous amount of water (ten glasses a day) reduces this risk. Protein *deficiency,* however, is vastly more common than overdose. Protein overdose would almost certainly require truly excessive reliance on protein supplements as total meal replacements.

from the lean. In fact, good health and nutrition depend on adequate protein.

This becomes even more important in a weight-training program when, during a workout, you disrupt the structure of muscle fibers in order to build stronger muscles.

Egg whites, nonfat yogurt, fat-trimmed meats, and fish give the highest protein efficiency ratio in a low-fat form. Egg whites are the champion of proteins—the most perfectly balanced, completely utilized protein on earth. About 96 percent of egg protein can be assimilated. Milk is next at about 60 percent. Then come the meats at roughly 40 percent, which is still considered "high quality." Vegetables vary, but up to 15 percent protein at best.

Forget these exact percentages, though, and just remember the protein concept. When various foods are combined into a meal, surplus amino acids from one food will combine with spare aminos from another food to form unexpected, complete proteins. So being overly precise about protein grams is utterly fruitless (so to speak).

If you're worried about "fattening," high-quality protein will prove invaluable to you and can be used to create such delicious low-fat dishes as an egg-white vegetable omelette and steamed lobster with lemon juice. Reduce the butter and oil, and substitute herbs, marinades, vinegars, and seasonings. In time you'll realize that the food itself is so flavorful it doesn't need the extra fat.

While some plants and vegetables—such as beans, brown rice, wild rice, and barley—contain some protein, they're not the best source of it for physically active people because they don't provide all the essential amino acids. (Protein is made of amino acids.) The nine "essential" ones must be contained in food because your body cannot manufacture them.

Vegetarian diets provide protein through specific combinations of carbohydrates containing complementary "incomplete proteins" that form a "complete" protein, with all nine essential aminos. Beans and corn, for example, contain incomplete proteins that combine to form a complete, usable protein.

While one gram of lean animal-based protein contains about five calories, the equivalent of one gram of lean vegetarian protein (e.g., beans with rice) contains about twenty-nine calories—80 percent of which come from carbohydrates. To meet your daily protein quota without overloading on carbohydrates, you'll need to rely on lean animal protein. (All animal protein sources have all of the essential amino acids.)

Early humans depended on vegetable staples, until the invention of new technologies—like the spear and the bow and arrow—made meat more plentiful. This new diet probably contributed to the increase in physical vigor of the race. Anthropologists say that this may explain why physiques from vegetarian populations are generally smaller and weaker than those from meat-eating societies.

BEST SOURCES OF GRAINS AND LEGUMES

Best Protein Sources*	Best Carbohydrate Sources
Soybeans	Brown rice
Split peas	Whole barley
Kidney beans	Whole buckwheat
Dried whole peas	Whole rye
Wheat germ	Foxtail millet
Lima beans	Wild rice
Black–eyed peas	Whole corn
Lentils	Pearl millet
Black beans	Whole wheat
Navy beans	Rolled oats

* Plant proteins do provide the body with resources for building muscle; however, they are not as readily available in maximum doses as animal proteins.

Source: *Optimum Sports Nutrition*, by Dr. Michael Colgan

At The FIRM, we maintain that protein needs are based on at least one gram for each two pounds of body weight—and more for athletes, especially when strength-training. This is about three to five servings each day. Build your meals around protein. If you weigh 130 pounds, your daily diet should include at least sixty-five grams of the proteins we mentioned above. If you have any type of increased activity level above sedentary, you need more. If you're involved in strenuous activity several times a week and work out with weights, your needs may be even higher—20–30 percent high-quality protein, or about 400–500 calories per 2,000-calorie day.

Many experts now agree that the USDA's Recommended Daily Allowance of .75 grams of protein per kilogram of body weight is strictly for the sedentary. Keep in mind that the RDA for protein is about 15 percent of daily calories. Protein requirements for a competitive natural bodybuilder can range from a daily low of 45 percent to a high of 70 percent.

Controlled studies conducted over the last decade indicate that increased athletic capacity requires increased protein consumption. Protein provides the bricks for rebuilding muscle and everything else with amino acids. If you are serious about building better health, you must include regular servings of high-quality, amino-acid complete, low-fat protein in *each* of your daily meals, including snacks.

We've observed many low-fat eaters at The FIRM who don't get the results they want because they also eat low protein. Lean muscle mass cannot be built with the wrong kind of calories. If you work out regularly and don't see results, your problems probably include skipping meals, especially breakfast, and a diet with too little protein and too much fat. Once again, protein should be included at regular intervals throughout the day; otherwise, your protein ratio will always be less than the required 25 percent of total daily calories.

Because the body cannot store protein, serious bodybuilders maintain a constant supply by eating small servings of lean protein (no more than twenty grams) every two hours throughout the day. (The liver converts excess protein into carbohydrate or fat, whichever the body needs most at the moment.) Along with the protein, a portion of complex carbohydrate must also be eaten in order to metabolize the protein quickly and repair the muscle tissues promptly.

If you think keeping up your protein while watching your weight is a challenge, you're not entirely wrong. First, it's true that most proteins come in a "package" loaded with fat. Second, it's almost impossible to get the necessary amount of protein to maximize your workout unless you use a meal replacement or carry a survival kit. In fact, after decades of extensive study, some experts conclude that athletes must use a supplement to get maximal protein intake.

At least 20–30 percent of daily caloric intake must be lean and complete protein to retain muscle while losing fat. To get the protein more easily, try using one protein meal replacement each day; it will give you the immediate benefit of filling you up with useful protein, carbohydrates, vitamins, and minerals—without the fat—and it is a great alternative to junk food or going hungry.

Meal substitutes usually come in the form of wafers or powders. Designed to help the body burn stored fat rather than muscle tissue, the meal substitutes work best for athletes striving for fat reduction with maximum muscular definition.

We have found the following meal substitutes particularly satisfactory:

PROTEIN POWDER (milk, egg, or soy-based proteins)

A protein supplement without carbohydrates, each serving can contain twenty to thirty grams of protein and about 150–200 calories. This is the lowest calorie source for complete proteins. Add fresh fruit, juice, or milk to complete the meal.

PROTEIN POWDER WITH CARBOHYDRATES (milk, soy, or soy-based protein with carbohydrate)

A meal replacement protein with carbohydrates, each serving can contain twenty to thirty grams of protein and about 250–350 calories. A higher calorie source for complete proteins, this can be mixed with water for a complete meal.

Each serving is equivalent to twenty (one gram), peptide-bonded, free amino-acid tablets or capsules.

If you're lactose intolerant, use a meal replacement drink based on egg whites and other amino acids. Soy-based protein powders are available for vegetarians and those with milk and egg allergies. However, because of soy-based products' lower Protein Efficiency Ratio (PER), more calories are required to achieve the same muscle-building effect as the animal-based supplements.

15–20 PERCENT NATURAL, UNPROCESSED FATS

Fats and oils are the least efficient forms of energy, but they prolong the digestive process and keep you feeling full from five to eight hours after a meal. That's one reason why Americans adore them. Fats and oils are present in some degree in all naturally occurring foods. Their essential nutrients are found only in fresh, mechanically pressed oils from nuts and seeds.

According to Dr. Udo Erasmus in his book *Fats That Heal, Fats That Kill,* beginning in about 1920, modern technology changed oil processing dramatically; prior to that healthful substances were not changed into what many experts are now recognizing as harmful substances. Virtually all liquid oils you buy at the supermarket have been extracted from seeds with the use of solvents (such as heptane, a type of gasoline), degummed, refined, bleached, and deodorized! Begun in 1911, the final step of oil processing, hydrogenation, turns liquid oils into cheap, spreadable products such as margarines and shortening. Used extensively in many baking goods and snack foods, hydrogenated and partially hydrogenated oils have recently been discovered to contain dangerous "trans-fatty acids."

According to statistics reported in 1979, Americans' consumption of fats and oils—an approximate and unbelievable 168 grams per day—was the highest in the world! It was also reported that Americans consumed about 40 percent of their calories in the form of fats. At 9 calories per gram, that's an incredible 1,512 calories daily, or close to 56 percent of the average daily caloric intake! When using the new "body mass index" standard, the latest figures show that the majority of Americans are officially overweight. Ironically, the cause of this obesity epidemic may well be the "low-fat diet." Since 1980, Americans have lowered their fat intake from 40 percent to 33 percent. That's good. But, according to recent USDA food consumption data, they've simultaneously increased their annual sugar intake from 120 pounds in 1970 to 150 pounds in 1995. That's awful. And since we know that the body turns refined sugars into fat, it's no secret why we're putting on weight.

Fats and oils don't have to be complicated. Use these three principles to include or exclude fats in your diet:

1. *Seek out the two essential unsaturated fatty acids (EFAs): linoleic acid and linolenic acid.* They are mandatory, hence the word "essential," for the total absence of these nutrients results in death! Deficiency symptoms include impaired growth and development of children, behavioral problems in children and adults, hair loss, heart and circulatory problems, impaired vision, and fertility problems. We need about 3 to 10 percent

SOPHIA FLOYD

AGE: 38
PROFESSION: EXECUTIVE SECRETARY,
SOUTH CAROLINA HOUSE OF REPRESENTATIVES

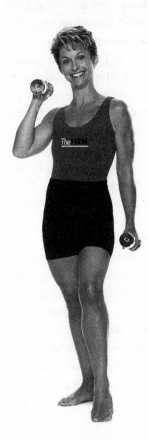

A small, stunningly dressed and immaculately groomed wife and mother of two boys, Sophia initially came to The FIRM because she wasn't happy with the way she looked. "I've been overweight before. I peaked at 140 in my teen years. I always wore baggy clothes and I wanted to be in things that were fitted."

Sophia is the first to admit that working out and teaching at The FIRM have given her enormous confidence as well as shapeliness and strength. "I feel like I look pretty good, and that comes across in everything I do."

She openly confesses to having had "scale obsession," weighing herself every day for ten years. "I was in a bad mood if the scales were up. If they were down, I was happy-go-lucky. But now I don't. I get on the scales every couple of months and I find that it's always the same. But I did not get to that point until I started coming here."

It's not just weight maintenance that keeps Sophia (and her husband, who works out at The FIRM religiously) coming back. "I'm teaching at 3:30 today, and I'm really excited about it because I want to move my body. I want to sweat. It's not because I want to go burn some calories because I overate or something—I want to move. I can't imagine what it would be like not to exercise!"

(continued)

SOPHIA'S TIPS FOR BEGINNERS:

○ Quit going on silly diets. You lose twenty, you gain back thirty. Just get your mind on basics and be sensible about what you put in your mouth.

○ Exercise four days a week.

○ If you're going to have pizza, have it, but eat one piece, not the whole thing.

○ Focus on your good body parts during a workout—if you have good legs, focus on them. If you've got a stomach that pokes out, stop looking at it.

○ You're not going to be happy with every single body part, so don't try.

○ Foodwise, if it comes from a tree or the ground, eat all you want, don't deprive yourself. But if it's fake or processed, I just don't think our bodies are equipped for it.

of our daily calories, or about 9 to 30 grams per day, of these specific oils. Look for them in raw nuts and seeds. Flax and pumpkin seeds are superior sources for both EFAs. Because flax seed has the additional benefit of improving intestinal elimination, many FIRM video leads and cast members have learned to include regular portions in their diets.

2. *Select fresh, unrefined seed oils.* While all other bottled fats may taste good, they do very little for your health or figure. For those times when you must use bottled oil, try virgin olive oil, the only oil widely available that is not heat-processed or refined. If it is not labeled virgin, it, too, has been through the same processing steps as the supermarket oils. Although virgin olive oil has only a small amount of one EFA, research shows that it protects against cardiovascular disease and may enhance brain function.

3. *Stop cooking in fat.* You don't need to fry or sauté all of your foods. For those times when you really must have a little fat for flavor, stick to the real things: Olive oil and butter are far superior to margarine and shortening.

When you follow our suggestions for eating low-fat foods, you'll automatically get the oils you need—and the figure you want!

FOOLPROOF STRATEGIES FOR LOWERING FAT

If you're like most people, your actual fat intake will surprise—not to say shock—you! We know many clients who began keeping a food diary with the assumption that they were healthy eaters, then couldn't believe the amount of fat they were consuming. Our advice to them was to reduce fat intake and simultaneously increase protein *asap!*

(Those of you who have The FIRM Personal Fitness CD-ROM can use the Food Data Base—the largest of its kind, containing 17,000 foods and their nutrient values—to plan your meals and manage your nutrition. The Smart Health Calendar allows you to immediately audit your past eating habits and improve your daily diet.)

Lowering your fat intake may seem difficult at first, but with experience, it'll become easier. You'll know off the top of your head that a tablespoon of olive oil contains *fourteen grams of fat*—practically your entire daily allowance. And you'll begin to recognize low-fat food from miles away. Here are some great tips for banishing unnecessary fat calories:

- Avoid packaged dishes, processed foods, and no-no snacks like potato chips and nachos.
- Use fresh cooking oils sparingly. Olive oil is our preference; store it in your refrigerator.
- Use nonfat dairy products.
- Use low-fat meats—nonfat turkey is preferred.
- Trim the visible fat from your meats whenever possible.
- Avoid sauces and salad dressings—use balsamic vinegar and/or lemon juice for a really tasty dressing alternative.
- Steam or dry-grill meats, without oil.
- Eliminate cheese from your diet—with the exception of a little parmesan for seasoning.
- *Pretend* there is no such thing as a dessert course.

"I have struggled with my weight all my life, and I just never thought I would have nice-looking legs. Well, they are well on their way; I can't wait to see what happens in the next twenty workouts. The FIRM is safe and it gives results; you feel stronger and more powerful. No other method has produced this."

CHERYL CARROLL, 37,
software systems engineer, Clairton, Pennsylvania

THE SKINNY ON FOOD SUPPLEMENTS

Physically active people need their vitamins! No one thinks twice about fertilizing plants to boost growth or about feeding farm animals nutrient-rich food loaded with vitamins and minerals to promote superior development. So why should humans be different?

Research cited in Colgan's *Optimum Sports Nutrition* continues to show that people who supplement their diets have a definite health advantage. Vitamins and minerals are extremely important, especially when restricting calories and building new muscle tissue—and they also prevent disease and delay aging!

The backbone of any supplemental program should include vitamins A, B, C, and E, and the minerals calcium, magnesium, zinc, and selenium.

It's a good idea to try out new supplements to see if they improve your health and well-being. For example: Vitamin C is a guaranteed immune system booster, and vitamin A and zinc can reduce skin eruptions. Keep in mind that it is often necessary to take supplements for three or four weeks to see an appreciable difference, especially since B and C are water soluble.

While using individual supplement capsules is generally recommended over combination tablets, the latter is more convenient. Some formulas are frequently low in specific vitamins and minerals and don't allow for special health needs. If you use a multiple vitamin, read the label and add individual substances where needed. Take the highest quality vitamin/mineral supplements, preferably in powdered form packed in clear gelatin capsules. Even the best of diets can be improved with the addition

TRACIE LONG

AGE: 30
PROFESSION: MANAGER, FIRM STUDIO,
CHARLESTON, SOUTH CAROLINA

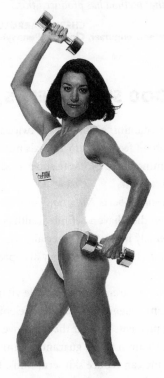

Considered by many the instructor's instructor, strong, warm, and confident, Tracie began at The FIRM as a client, became an instructor, and was soon promoted to full-time staff trainer—in which role she has been preparing instructors since 1991.

Tracie originally started The FIRM workouts because of a weight problem. "The first time I tried to lose weight was years ago when I was in school," she recalls. "Not knowing much about dieting, I did the Slimfast diet for a week. I was really grouchy and had a headache all the time."

Then she took a nutrition class and learned to change her eating behaviors. She immediately cut fat from her diet and began to keep a food diary. "I have always had to exercise more than the average person," she explains, "but changing my lifestyle and diet made all the exercise results apparent."

When she was chosen from seventy instructors to lead both *The Tortoise* and *The Hare* videos, Tracie knew she was in for a challenge. Because video makes you look heavier, she had to go 20 pounds below her natural weight in nine weeks! "Once the video was over," she admits, "some of the weight came back. I'm most comfortable a little heavier than my best 'video weight.' Now that I'm more experienced at eating correctly, I'm able to maintain my weight at only 5 to 8 pounds over that ideal."

(continued)

Still, seeing her commit to a goal and stick to it had a positive effect on her future husband. "I think this determination rubbed off on him," she smiles. "He started setting goals for himself and following through with them. He also started to eat better and train with weights. I also think it made him want to marry me."

Tracie is able to maintain her motivation because, as she says, "When I was heavier (141 pounds), I was also depressed. I wore baggy clothes and was always uncomfortable. Now I wear whatever I want and feel good about it. I have developed a healthy understanding of what my body needs. When food is a major issue in your life, all you look forward to is eating. Now I only eat when my body tells me to!"

TRACIE'S TIPS FOR BEGINNERS:

- Keep a food diary; you'll know how much you've eaten and can better evaluate your hunger levels and decide if you really need "food energy" or just want to nibble.
- Eat only when you are hungry.
- Survival kits of food (see chapter 4) are the ticket to successful weight loss. They help you transfer junk food cravings to more healthy substitutes.
- Eat three servings of fruit per day and drink lots of water; they keep the energy level up, so you eat fewer starchy carbs.
- If you slip up, just say "It's okay," and move on; don't let a lapse turn into a three-day binge.

of basic nutrients. What follows are suggested vitamins and minerals for athletes (Colgan, as above; M. Tanny, *Bodybuilding Nutrition*; C. Sheats, *Lean Bodies*) (Note: IU = international units; 3.3IU = 1 RE or Retinol Equivalents).

Oil Soluble Vitamins—A, D, and E

If not taken at the right levels, vitamins and minerals are potent and can adversely affect health. They must also be taken in the correct ratio of one to another. Oil-based vitamins, including A, D, and E, are stored in body fat and can be toxic when used to excess. Correct dosage levels are extremely important.

- *Vitamin A (Retinol):* To prevent deficiency, the Recommended Daily Allowance for vitamin A is 5,000 IU (1,000–2,000 RE) for adults, but many experts believe this amount is too low. Numerous studies have shown widespread vitamin A deficiency in both athletes and the general public. If you want to bolster your body's store of A, eat foods such as liver, carrots, beets, greens, spinach, broccoli, yellow fruits, and yellow vegetables.

  Vitamin A, which aids in the repair and growth of body tissue and in the maintenance of soft, healthy skin, may help control acne and other skin problems. It is also considered to have an anticancer effect, especially the beta carotene form—which functions mainly as an antioxidant and is not toxic—found in the aforementioned vegetables and fruit. You'll need to take *both* the vitamin A and beta carotene forms since the latter has a low rate of conversion to true vitamin A. If you are physically active and/or experience daily eyestrain, consider increasing your dosage to between 3,000–15,000 IU per day.
- *Vitamin D:* This vitamin is essential to the body's ability to absorb calcium. Although we can manufacture D through exposure to the sun, supplementation has become necessary because of the now-acknowledged hazards of suntanning. Cod liver oil is one of the best sources of D, especially for young children, teens, and pregnant women.
- *Vitamin E:* E has proven to be an aid to cardiovascular health because of its role on the cellular respiration of all muscles, including cardiac and skeletal. Take about one hundred to four hundred IU daily (check the label for content), using the natural d-alpha form of the vitamin, which is resistant to rancidity. Unprocessed fresh wheat germ is an excellent source of E, as are fish oils.

Water Soluble Vitamins—B and C

The B vitamins, combined with C, are powerful stress inhibitors and useful energy boosters. Water soluble vitamins are available to nourish cells for a short time and are excreted through the urine. Ideally, each of your meals should contain a food source like broccoli or kale for vitamins B and C.

- *Vitamin B:* Vitamin B complex, which includes vitamins B1, B2, B3 (niacin), B5, B6, B9 (folic acid), and B12, is found in red meats and unprocessed grains. It is essential for a healthy nervous system. Stress can deplete B, so you want to include foods high in it, such as vegetables, fresh, clean fruits, whole grains, and meats at every meal. It is difficult to get enough vitamin B complex on a daily basis, so it is best to take supplements to ensure optimal intake for optimal health.

   Many emotional problems in adults can be a result of a B complex deficiency. Eye tics, racing thoughts, disturbed sleep, and burning feet are all possible symptoms. Folic acid is especially important for pregnant women, to aid in the prevention of birth defects.
- *Vitamin C:* Found in fresh fruits and vegetables, C is a powerful aid in fighting injury and illness. It boosts the immune system and strengthens the body on a cellular level; unsightly bruises indicate a need for additional C and citrus bioflavonoids. Many nutritionists recommend high levels of vitamin C, ranging from 1,000 mg–2,000 mg a day. Space your dosage over the course of the day. For example, if your total dosage is 1,000 mg/day, take 500 mg in the morning and 500 mg at night.

Minerals

These six minerals are particularly necessary for athletes and are often deficient from most Americans' diets:

- *Calcium and Magnesium:* These two minerals are essential to maximize bone mass, yet the average American's daily calcium intake is 743 mg—a figure way below the RDA of 1,200 mg. Pregnant and lactating women, young children, and teens may require as much as 2,000 mg per day. Athletes may require more than normal because bone mineralization increases tremendously in response to exercise stress. If your body doesn't contain enough calcium, it will cannibalize the skeleton to make up the difference. Leg cramps, which may indicate deficiencies, are caused by low levels of the companion mineral, magnesium. Magnesium is also especially important for health of the nervous system, and along with calcium and vitamin D, it aids in better sleep and better dispositions!

Women have to be particularly mindful of calcium to prevent osteoporosis, but two out of three women don't get enough of it. Since most women avoid dairy products and drink coffee or tea, which inhibit calcium absorption, calcium and magnesium may be their most important mineral supplements.

To best use your calcium and magnesium, the body must also have adequate supplies of silicon, zinc, fluoride, copper, boron, manganese, phosphorous, and vitamin D. Boron improves calcium metabolism and utilization.

- *Selenium/Chromium:* These trace minerals seem to contribute to fighting body fat and building lean body mass. Chromium regulates blood sugar and helps to control the urge to eat sweets. Daily selenium should be taken in a 3:1 ratio with chromium. Most multiple formulas are equally balanced: If you don't take a multiple formula, consider buying additional selenium to meet the 3:1 ratio.
- *Zinc:* This trace mineral, which also helps control skin problems, is best consumed with food; zinc gluconate and zinc picolinate are the forms most easily absorbed. Athletes have an increased zinc requirement because excessive sweating can cause a loss of as much as 3 mg of zinc per day.
- *Iron:* Inadequate iron is a common mineral deficiency in the U.S. population as a whole (Colgan, Sheats) and for athletes in particular. Iron is much more easily absorbed from meat than from vegetable sources. While spinach seems like a good option, your body takes in only about 1.4 percent of its iron, as opposed to 20 percent from beef. Often overlooked sources of iron include pork liver, beef liver, farina, raw clams and oysters, dried peaches, egg yolks, nuts, asparagus, molasses, and oatmeal.

While you can get iron from beans, raisins, tomato juice, and red meat, research shows that even moderate levels of exercise can drain your iron stores, especially if you're a menstruating female and/or borderline anemic. Heavy coffee or tea drinkers also need extra iron. Find out from your physician if you're anemic or borderline anemic before taking iron supplements because a person may have too little or too much. Be careful!

DEAR FIRM

"I used to work out three to five hours a day when I was trying to lose a great deal of weight (I realize now that was crazy). With The FIRM I realize that as long as I concentrate and put my best into each exercise, I don't have to kill myself to get results. No other method effectively streamlines hamstrings and buttocks to perfection."

**LORIE B., 21,
human resources manager, Groveport, Ohio**

Now that we've run through the nutritional basics of FIRM Fuel, we'd like to share with you Six Simple Ways to Reshape Your Body Faster.

THE FAB SIX

1. Upgrade Your Fuel: Your goal should be to build radiant, vibrant health, and to have abundant energy, a healthy complexion, and a pleasant disposition. All of this comes from eating excellent food at frequent intervals every day. Eliminate alcohol and sugars, and remember to keep blood sugar levels high with small, frequent high-quality meals and snacks. This helps greatly in controlling those terrible urges that lead us to bingeing, overeating, and destroying all of our hard work.

2. Eat Three Healthy Meals a Day, Plus Two Protein-Rich Snacks: People who eat very few calories can have high water retention in the tissues. High water retention creates the illusion of being overweight, but it can be a sign of malnutrition, so take care of yourself!

3. Practice Portion Control: Any food becomes fattening if you eat too much of it!

4. More Muscle, Less Fat: That's what's accomplished by combining The FIRM workouts with FIRM Fuel!

5. Increase Activity: The more you work out, the more fat you burn, especially when you're not adding to the fat supply with a deadly food regimen!

6. Learn FIRM Rules to go with your new life!

FIRM RULES

Looks Don't Lie

Your body advertises everything you put in your mouth. It stands to reason that if you're overweight, you eat foods that are low in nutrients and high in fat. If you're slim and toned, you almost certainly consume high-energy, low-fat fuel. If you are chronically tired and moody, you probably aren't giving your body top-quality fuel. If you think nobody will know about that candy bar, you're wrong. You may as well glue it on your hips!

Notice what professional trainers and professional athletes eat. Chicken breast, no skin. An orange. Salad. Protein drinks. These people understand the whole picture. They're toned, lean, pure muscle, not only because they work out, but because they appreciate the difference between high energy, low-fat foods and their opposites.

What You May Be Doing Wrong

Most people don't feel like exercising, even though they know they should. We have a strong suspicion that their low energy comes from low-quality body fuel. No wonder they don't feel like working out. In addition to trying to diet without exercise, look to these common culprits for lack of success:

- not eating on a regular basis throughout the day
- too many high-fat dietary staples such as mayonnaise, peanut butter, and whole milk
- too many heat-treated refined fats in fried foods, packaged breads, commercial foods, entrees, and desserts

- too many hydrogenated fats such as margarine spreads
- not enough protein
- not enough raw, fresh, fibrous, complex carbohydrates
- underestimating the quantities you consume, especially snack foods, sauces, salad dressings, sugared beverages, and fruit drinks
- too many high-fat calories
- too many low-quality processed, refined foods
- not meeting the Recommended Daily Allowance for vitamins and minerals, based on the needs of sedentary individuals
- not getting the right fats—two essential fatty acids are critical for health

Learning How to Eat Right with a Food Diary

You know by now that the best diet for optimal athletic health is low in fat, high in complex carbohydrates and fiber, and that it contains at least one gram of protein per two pounds of body weight. Here is the question you should ask yourself every time you eat: "Are the calories I'm eating of the highest possible nutritional value and the lowest fat content?"

One of the most effective ways of doing that is by keeping a food diary and listing every single thing you put in your mouth every day. One of the goals of this diary will be to help you achieve and maintain a well-toned body by consuming clean foods. Keep a positive, aggressive mindset. You *can* change. A diet of natural foods and exercise is the path to better physical and mental health. If you're on an improved diet, you'll see exercise results much faster.

What to Do When Eating Out

Try to select a place that has a buffet. If this is not an option, order dry-grilled chicken breast, if possible, steamed vegetables, and potato, rice, or pasta. If you have to substitute other foods, keep as close to your ideal as possible. Whatever you do, don't let the chef add any sauce, and don't be bullied by your friends into falling off the chow wagon. And definitely don't let the waiter show you the dessert tray!

Simplify Kitchen Techniques

Make a simple, pure art form out of preparing your food. Steam chicken or turkey breasts. If necessary, make muffins, bread, rice, or potatoes for the following day. Plan to spend some time each evening chopping and storing vegetables and fruits. Collect knives. Become a connoisseur of the best tools.

Order Bulk Carbohydrates

To save money buy whole grains in ten-pound lots wholesale from your health food store. Complex carbs are one place you can save significant dollars. Invest in plenty of plastic-top containers.

Buy the Best Appliances

Use an automatic rice steamer and experiment with different rice types. One of our favorites is a mixture of wild and brown rice, but feel free to experiment, adding flavor with soy sauce and sea salt.

Another important accessory is a top quality vegetable slicer, handy for carrots and potatoes.

Replace Fats with Herbs

A handful of fresh herbs (or a teaspoonful if you must use dried) sprinkled liberally over your proteins and carbs makes a plain dish infinitely more flavorful, even exotic. Garlic and onion are essential for low-fat flavor, but also experiment with sage, basil, thyme, tarragon, curry, chili powders, and the many more unique, organic flavor powerhouses. Also, think about starting your own herb garden!

Make Superior Choices for Clean, Simple Meals

Just because your revised menus are good for you doesn't mean they can't be scrumptious as well. With garlic, herbs, and a judicious use of olive oil, your meals can be highly nutritious and delightfully pleasing to the eye and palate. Here are some outstanding examples of this truth:

1. FISH
   Fresh fillet with lemon and herbs
   Steamed dark leafy greens with sesame seeds
   Baked squash
   Baked potato with garlic

2. SIRLOIN
   Fat-trimmed ground meat with garlic and fresh ginger
   Rice with mushrooms
   Green beans and broccoli
   Raw beets and carrots

3. OMELETTE
   Three egg whites, one egg yolk with spring onion
   Whole grain cereal
   Orange or other fruit in season

4. SEAFOOD
   Scallops steamed with fresh dill and garlic
   Stir-fried dark leafy greens with mushrooms
   Whole wheat pasta with fresh tomatoes and a touch of Parmesan

5. CHICKEN
   Baked skinless breast with fresh thyme and oregano
   Boiled potatoes with sesame seed and garlic
   Raw carrots and raisins
   Watercress with mixed lentil sprouts

6. NONFAT YOGURT
   Nonfat yogurt
   Fresh pineapple

Raw mixed lentil sprouts
Sweet potato with Nutrasweet and cinnamon

7. BEANS & RICE
Rice cakes
Fat-free pinto bean spread
Raw carrot
Apple or orange

8. TURKEY
Stir-fried breast strips with garlic and onions
Stir-fried spinach
Green beans and red pepper
Brown rice and fresh raw corn medley

Make a beautiful presentation on a lovely plate, and you'll love eating healthy!

Don't Leave Home Without a Portable Survival Kit

It's hard to withstand temptation, so you have to be prepared to resist foods that will defeat your goals. One way to tackle this problem is by developing the habit of carrying a "survival kit" with you at all times. It should include water, since water is one of your best defenses against hunger. Carry a refillable twelve- to sixteen-ounce jug every day, and drink whenever you feel hungry.

Load up the rest of your survival kit with ten to twenty grams of non-fat protein and several servings of fresh fruit or other fibrous carbohydrates. Include a paring knife, plastic forks, and spoons.

Save your survival kit for your weakest moments, when you really need it. Don't eat from it all day, especially if you're not really hungry. Use it only when tempted by high-fat food, not when you're bored sitting in traffic or hungry because you missed your 2 P.M. snack. Following are six examples of survival kits that do the trick:

1. 3¹/₂ ounces water-packed tuna
   carrots, celery
   1 orange
   2 rice cakes
2. 8 ounces nonfat, sugar-free yogurt
   12 raisins
   1 banana
3. 3 amino wafers
   1 cold baked sweet potato
4. 3–4 ounces chopped turkey or chicken breast
   low-fat mustard
   homemade low-fat bread or pancake
   celery (optional)
5. 3–4 ounces homemade tuna salad (made with dill pickle, yogurt, and
   homemade mayonnaise)
   fat-free, yeast-free rye crackers
   1 apple
6. blender drink made with:
   1 scoop (20 grams) vanilla protein powder
   1 pack Nutrasweet or 1 teaspoon sugar
   6 ice cubes
   10 fresh strawberries
   1 teaspoon vanilla
   4 ounces water/skim milk/yogurt

Resist Food Triggers

According to Stephen P. Gullo, Ph. D., in *Thin Tastes Better,* eating triggers are the things that remind us to eat. We have to be aware of these triggers in order to control them. Here are some examples:

- FOOD
  - cooking and preparing food
  - seeing and smelling foods

- EMOTIONS
  - work or social stress
  - ravenous, out-of-control hunger
  - loneliness
  - depression
  - anxiety, fear of failure
  - boredom
- EVENTS
  - parties or social events with fancy luxury foods
  - friends who eat with abandon
  - habitual meal times

Tell yourself that you will not eat in response to an eating trigger every time you come in contact with one. Factors such as feeling lonely or depressed, or feeling that you deserve a treat, are not reasons to eat. Don't give in! Find and use other rewards besides food.

In your food diary, make a list of your "failure foods"—the ones for which you have a personal weakness: If you eat one, you'll eat one hundred. Scan the list constantly and, when confronted with temptation, say this mantra to yourself: "These are the foods I cannot eat in moderation. They ruin my figure, and, therefore, are poison to me."

Also write down the specific emotions that trigger a food binge and practice saying this mantra: "I am identifying the emotional states that make me eat. The ordinary human feelings of loneliness, anger, boredom, and depression are common culprits that will not steal my resolve." By so doing, you'll learn to dissociate these feelings from eating and to substitute healthier behaviors.

Next, make a record of the events that trigger food binges—whether stress or depression. Say this mantra: "Daily problems do not rule my existence. I will have a life outside my problems, and I will not eat when these problems invariably surface."

Prevent Relapse

Maintaining a new diet is the greatest challenge that any person faces when changing her or his health habits. Everyone will slip once in a while, but the trick is to respond constructively to a lapse before it compels you to give up. The following are suggestions that may help you in breaking the slip-fall-give up cycle:

1. Identify high-risk situations.
2. Outlast the urge to give up.
3. If you have slipped, don't blame yourself. Analyze the situation, learn the cause, and be prepared the next time the trigger appears.
4. Enlist the help of a friend. It's helpful to associate with like-minded friends when you are struggling for positive food habits. Less disciplined friends can urge you to indulge, and destroy your best intentions.

Anna's classic trouble zone is after work when she's tired. There's no food ready to eat, she has more work to do, and her two boys are hungry. So it's easy to slip, especially if she hasn't eaten for the past six hours. Low blood sugar and fatigue spell b-i-n-g-e because sugar becomes the sole preoccupation of a starving mind in search of a quick fix. To prevent this, Anna's mantra is "Never go too long without high-quality fuel." She finds meal replacement drinks are perfect for binge control. That mantra is so simple, yet so crucial.

Self-Affirmation: Learn to Turn Negative Thoughts Positive

Many people have to acquire a positive workout and dietary attitude. Thoughts, both negative and positive, can become self-fulfilling prophecies. Your mind and your thoughts are powerful: If you believe something's true, then it is. For example, if you believe you're a failure when it comes to weight loss, you'll never achieve your maximum potential.

However, if you train yourself to refocus negative into positive, you'll have the power to do anything you choose. The trick is to stop yourself each time you are about to indulge in a negative thought and to replace it with a positive one. For instance, turn

- "I'll never get rid of this extra weight" into "I can learn to eat correctly and exercise."
- "I can't control my eating" into "I can learn to exert control."
- "I probably won't keep a food diary" into "The food diary will help me tremendously."
- "I hate the way I look" into "People look at me and see a healthy person."

Now that you've studied The FIRM Rules, we're going to wrap up with the absolute essentials for reaching your goal.

DEAR FIRM

"Throw away your cellulite creams, ladies! There is no extra fat on my body and, since The FIRM, no cellulite! I've had it since age fifteen, lost it at twenty. The FIRM has changed my life by giving me a great body, a sound mind, and great self-esteem; and I feel so strong."

NATALIE K., 25,
receptionist, Brooklyn, New York

THE SEVEN KEYS TO FIRM SUCCESS

I. Identify and Eliminate Problem Foods

Firm resolve is essential here because you probably love your poisons. In fact, your body could crave the very foods that give you allergies or skin or gastrointestinal problems. Through observation and self-knowledge, learn to avoid them. Identify and eliminate these foods, and your body will thank you.

Through your food diary, you'll be able to identify trouble-making foods by charting your reaction to them and noticing the way they make you feel. On days when you have trouble with elimination, are bloated, or feel lethargic, note the foods you've eaten. Look for patterns. Many gastrointestinal problems can be solved by eliminating sweet carbohydrates with a high glycemic index.

To cure common intestinal problems, eliminate:

- simple sugars
- dairy products containing lactose, such as milk and yogurt
- grains containing glutens, such as wheat, oats, rye, and barley

Test for these common allergies:

- yeast (in breads, crackers, nutritional supplements, beer, and wine)
- sulfates (preservatives used in canned goods, such as tomatoes and red wine)
- eggs
- corn
- milk
- soy products
- wheat

II. Drink Lots of Water

Drink water, water, and more water! It's great for you! Optimally, you should strive to take in eight to ten eight-ounce glasses a day. That's at least four sixteen-ounce bottles a day. This does not include colas, coffee, tea, fruit juice, or diet drinks. Water alone flushes out waste products and helps fill you up when you're hungry. And you may just find that your skin looks and feels healthier as well!

III. Sugar Has to Be Off-Limits

It's hard to believe how many people eat sugar all day long. Some do M&Ms. Others chew piece after piece of bubble gum just to get the juice. Believe us, these are baaaad habits! No amount of heredity can make up for this type of abuse. After eating sweets, the blood sugar "high" immediately plummets to an even lower level than it was prebinge. In addition, refined sugar encourages your body to keep fat stored. You have no room in your diet for empty calories. Out, out, damned sugar!

IV. Alcohol and Other No-No's

Youth can make us feel invincible. Many young athletes continue to use alcohol and other drugs, even though they work out regularly. This defeats the purpose of the workout! As people mature, they usually learn to reduce or give up habits that sabotage their health.

Alcohol has empty calories and no nutritional value. Two eight-ounce glasses of wine per day equal four hundred calories; this translates into approximately three pounds of weight-gain per month unless you add forty minutes of steady exercise daily to your routine or eliminate the same quantity of nutrient-dense food. Additionally, it isn't just the calories in alcohol that can make you fat. Research shows that alcohol reduces the body's normal fat-burning rate by one third; it is metabolized as a sugar, causing your blood sugar level to rise. It's no secret then that daily drinkers usually carry extra body fat.

On a restricted diet, you have no room for valueless food. If you indulge, try to limit yourself to one serving of alcohol. If you drink more than that, recover by taking extra vitamin B and C, and drink plenty of water. If you work out, water is especially important to prevent dehydration.

As women age, caffeinated beverages like coffee may cause a significant decline in bone density. This decrease augments the risk of hip and other bone fractures. Milk helps combat this bone loss, but reports indicate that the more coffee women drink, the less milk they consume. In addition to ingesting additional calcium supplements, put the mineral to use with a strength-training program. Remember the most significant, measurable improvements in bone density occur through regular weight lifting.

Daily regular use of nicotine, caffeine, alcohol, and other habitual drugs destroys energy, diminishes intelligence, and dampens creativity. These substances don't help solve problems, they exacerbate them. Living a good life is a challenge for all of us; you never regain lost days and opportunities. If you have a desire to indulge in unhealthy habits, it may be that you need to change your circle of friends or join a support group to help you find a healthier lifestyle. Make a decision to grow in a positive way, and use exercise to help you see that you can do it and do it well.

V. Don't Fall Off the Wagon

Be aware of diet sabotage. Remind yourself that any body composition change is difficult, especially the last five or ten pounds. Enjoy well-earned compliments, but don't let them make you complacent. Stick with your program. And if you do succumb to temptation, forgive yourself and get back on track. Remember, this is a diet for life, and you want to stay lean and strong as a panther. Congratulate yourself when you have a successful weigh-in, but don't lose sight of your long-term goals: more energy, a higher self-concept, and a healthier lifestyle.

DEAR FIRM

"I had succumbed to the idea that no amount of exercise would produce 'visible results' for a forty-three-year-old, especially someone with 'fat genes.' I told myself I would be happy with a healthy heart and a lumpy, completely ordinary body (lumpier after two cesareans). I was resigned forever to giving up short skirts, sleeveless dresses, or anything defining the waistline.

"But in the last eighteen months The FIRM has really reshaped my body. My hips are sleek for the first time in my life. My legs look longer, even if they are not. My upper arms don't jiggle, my shoulders are defined and shapely, and my waist looks smaller. I wear clothes that I thought were permanently out of my league. By the way, my husband loves my new body, too."

LYNDA K. B., 43,
English professor, Williamstown, Massachusetts

VI. Become a Sophisticated Eater

Make a conscious decision not to eat when a trigger arises. Going without dessert may bring a pang of loss, and what's worse, you may not be re-

ANNA'S "KICK COFFEE" MORNING PICK-UP DRINK

After having been a heavy coffee drinker for almost twenty years, Anna has been able to eliminate the habit with the help of her "Pick-Up Drink." All people are in need of immediate food in the morning after a night's fast. All too frequently, coffee is used as a "food substitute," since it quickly (however falsely) elevates blood sugar levels.

The danger of this practice is the inevitable rapid falling of blood sugar levels, which increases the craving for more caffeine and other quick sources of "energy," such as sugar and other empty carbohydrates. The key to success control (with this and other unhealthy habits such as alcohol abuse) is the use of high-density, high-value foods.

Dieters who attempt to control daily caloric levels are in the greatest danger of cheating between 3 P.M. and 7 P.M., when blood sugar levels are at their lowest. Our drink is low in calories, high in nutrients, and may be successfully incorporated into a weight-loss program. Used twice daily—once in the morning and again in the late afternoon—it should help you through the "no caffeine, low-calorie blues."

This type of drink is an excellent energy source for morning workouts, and it should be followed, as should all workouts, with a protein-rich meal with plenty of complex carbohydrates. It provides iron, B-vitamins, protein, minerals, digestive enzymes, and unrefined carbohydrates. Coffee, in contrast, robs the body of B-vitamins and minerals (especially calcium) and destroys digestive enzymes. Try to free yourself of the coffee habit!

THE FIRM PICK-UP DRINK

1 T. blackstrap molasses
1/2 t. yeast flakes
1/2 t. bee pollen
1/4 cup raw milk
hot water
1/2 T. calcium/magnesium mineral supplements

(This can be made in a blender or served over ice. Add digestive aids if you experience gas or intestinal bloating: HCl and/or pepsin-containing aids) warded for your effort until the fat layer on your body begins to melt away. You have to be able to discipline yourself to focus on the final goal. Discipline demands perseverance, and perseverance is the ability to follow through after the enthusiasm and emotion that started your resolution have passed.

VII. Master the Difference Between Appetite and Hunger

Learn to cruise on a half-full tank of fuel. As you change your diet, the "full" feeling you previously associated with satisfaction will change to a leaner, cleaner, lighter feeling. Don't be fooled by thinking the "full" feeling is your goal. When you switch to low-fat meals, you'll get hungry again much faster, but you'll also learn to maintain your blood sugar levels. Many people come to like not feeling full—they report having more energy all day long. Your body is able to maintain stable blood sugar levels throughout the day by eating five to six small meals.

Also learn to identify degrees of hunger. Slight hunger is good, but ravenous hunger can be disastrous and lead to bingeing. Prevent ruining your daily program by taking in *quality* fuel at regular intervals throughout the day. You cannot be lean and strong unless you eat regularly and correctly.

Most of us cycle between two states: starving and bingeing. Many people start the day with a breakfast pastry and coffee. Their blood sugar goes sky high—the first spike on their daily blood sugar graph. When blood sugar escalates too quickly, it takes a dive downward within a couple of hours. Mentally unable to focus and ravenously hungry, the low blood sugar victim then attacks a vending machine for more sweets and hits the second blood sugar spike of the day, followed by another blood sugar crash. For many, this destructive daily cycle continues until "happy hour," when alcohol becomes the blood sugar booster of choice.

When blood sugar zooms up and down, mood and concentration suffer. We feel stressed, anxious, irritable, and frustrated by the world. And once the daily vicious cycle of spikes and crashes begins, it's difficult to stabilize blood sugar levels later in the day. Without a sensible breakfast, the productive day you planned is all but over.

For long-term weight maintenance, we must eat when we have the need (every two to three hours throughout the day), but resist when we have only the desire (at the food table of a party). Hunger is the need to eat, while appetite is only the desire to eat. Don't think of hunger as an extreme condition associated with a growling stomach. Learn to associate hunger with brain function: The first symptom of hunger occurs when your thoughts roll slightly "out of focus." During the early stages of a blood sugar slump, a modest balanced snack will restore mental clarity in minutes. If you don't restore blood sugar soon enough, the resulting hunger attack may drive you to a sugar snack. Avoid triggering your appetite (and the possibility of a binge) by "grazing" throughout the day.

The foolproof method is to eat "by the clock"—every two to three hours. (Many people are so sensitive to blood sugar fluctuations that they function well only when they eat something every two hours.) To maximize your control over eating:

- Try not to skip any of the recommended meals.
- Never go with an empty stomach to functions where food is being served.
- Always carry survival food so you don't binge.
- Include complete protein in every meal.

When you skip meals, you often compensate by consuming too many calories later. You may think you've saved some calories from prior meals, but your body can only digest so much at one time. The excess may be stored as fat. Each of your meals must contain some kind of complete protein; this will give you the staying power you're missing from reduced fat levels.

You should prepare for workouts by eating a combination of simple and complex carbos about sixty to ninety minutes prior to the session. This will ensure that you have enough energy.

If you feel the need to burn extra fat calories, do it while you sleep! Try not to eat anything after 7 P.M., or five hours before going to bed.

"I lost fifteen pounds in three months of using The FIRM workouts, lost three inches from my waist, and had a tremendous boost in energy. Now, after seven months, I have lost forty pounds and six inches from my waist in total! Thank you!"

DARLA A. UMEMOTO, 30,
litigation specialist, Corona, California

GROW YOUNG WITH US

It really doesn't matter whether you're eighteen or eighty; there's always room for regeneration and revitalization in anybody's life. We at The FIRM feel strongly that the right kind of workout, the right kind of diet, and a sensible, moderate lifestyle will keep you at the height of your powers indefinitely. So if you're eighteen, you'll be laying the foundation for energy and health all through your life; and if you're eighty, you'll regain a vitality you thought was lost forever. Staying young or growing younger is entirely up to you!

CHAPTER 5

FIRM
bodies

O kay. Now that you've mastered the essentials of The FIRM methodology, nutritional plan, and lifestyle, you're ready for your workout, which begins with The FIRM BASIC DAILY DOZEN.

YOUR MUSCLES AND
HOW THEY'RE WORKED

Without learning how the classic weight training muscle isolation exercises work, you really don't have a clue about exercise. So here goes:

Your body contains some 639 muscles, which comprise 30 to 50 percent of your body weight. (More muscle is better.) Because the configuration of muscles is identical in men and women, the same exercises work for both sexes. In the upper body, men are about twice as strong as women.

Because you have large and small muscle groups, you need large and small dumbbells to tone them. (One way to spot a bogus exercise program: Only one size dumbbell is used.)

The most famous muscle in the body is the *biceps,* which lets you hold a grocery bag without dropping it. Muscles work in opposing pairs for flexion (the *biceps)* and extension (the *triceps):* The biceps contracts to bend the elbow. The triceps contracts to straighten the elbow.

The *biceps* muscle is isolated by the *biceps curl.* To isolate the muscle, keep the elbows in tight and the back straight, so you don't cheat by swinging the weight up with your back.

A firm *triceps* shapes the back of the upper arm. It is worked by the *french press* (elbows in and stationary) and by *triceps kickbacks* (elbows in and stationary).

The forearm muscles control the grip and wrist movement. They're worked automatically by holding the dumbbell.

If you ever need to punch an attacker, you need strong *pectorals*, which give men manly chests and women lovely breast support. (The breast itself is a gland and cannot be developed with exercise.) *Pectorals* and *triceps* are worked by *push-ups*.

Straight *crunches* work the *upper abdominals*. *Twisting crunches* work the *abdominal obliques*. The *lower abdominals* are worked by *leg pulleys* and by *reverse crunches*.

On the front of the thighs are the *quadriceps*. *Lunges* work the *quads*, as do *squats*. People with problem knees should do lunges and squats cautiously. These exercises will strengthen knees, if you don't do them too deeply in the beginning.

Outer thigh muscles are called *leg abductors* because they steal away (or abduct) the leg from the axis of the body. Inner thigh *adductors* return (or add) the leg to the axis of the body. *Leg lifts* with the top leg work the abductors. *Leg lifts* with the bottom leg work the adductors.

The *hamstrings* (aka *leg biceps*) on the back of the thigh are worked by various moves in *table position*. On all exercises, slight angle changes are used to work different areas of the muscles.

The *gluteus maximus* is the big muscle that gives you tight buttocks. Exercises for beautiful glutes include *bridgework* and *squats*, but the best exercises are *lunges* and the *tall-box leg press*.

Many clients tell us they dislike lunges more than any other exercise. It is difficult to do them with perfect form, and yet all clients agree that nothing gives them firmer fannies faster than lunges and tall-box step-ups. The exercises you dislike most are usually the ones you need most.

With The FIRM's *tall-box leg press*, we unknowingly reinvented a powerful technique used by Olympic athletes behind the iron curtain. This one exercise shapes beautiful *gluteal* muscles (buttocks), *quadriceps*, and leg *biceps*—all in absolutely perfect proportion! (A very tall fourteen-inch height works well for most exercisers.)

Short-box stepping (eight- to ten-inch height) has an *entirely different effect* from the tall-box leg press: The short box (familiar to step training classes) gives a low-impact *aerobic* effect. That's all. The tall box gives a powerful *muscle-shaping* effect. Step training was once hyped as the lower body solution, but it isn't. The short step shapes only the quadriceps, and only slightly.

Several movements work the *spinal erectors* that run up your backbone. If the spinal erectors aren't properly stretched and strengthened, low back pain results. Abdominal exercises also help the problematic low-back area. If you have back trouble, begin cautiously on spinal erector moves.

These big back muscles are the *latissimus dorsi* that give bodybuilders that distinctive V-shaped torso because they are also seen from the front when developed. *Bent-over rows* with *heavy* dumbbells work the lats, and make the waist appear smaller. The big diamond-shaped muscle at the back of the neck is the *trapezius*. It is worked with *shoulder rolls* using *heavy* dumbbells, and by *bent-over flys*.

Read this section with care and cross-reference it with the actual Daily Dozen exercises for optimal benefit.

THE DAILY DOZEN

FIRM BASICS, which should be done with weights every other day, are designed to work the twelve major muscles of your body. Doing them religiously will produce visible results, as you reshape your body proportionally. You should do all twelve of the exercises sequentially without resting between sets. Perform twelve to twenty repetitions of each exercise and repeat the cycle three times. Allow thirty minutes daily for the whole routine. However, before you begin, study the preceding section on the muscles in your body. Understanding what you're doing always enhances the enjoyment and efficacy of any workout.

Equipment

While many of the Daily Dozen can be performed using no equipment, you soon will want a basic set of equipment to maximize your results.

Equipment consists of (1) a set of dumbbells, (2) a tall step (approximately fourteen inches tall), (3) a dowel, and (4) a two- by four-inch board. If you can't find this generic equipment in your store, see the product list at the end of this book.

In all of these exercises, you should exhale on the lift and inhale on the release. Remember, don't hold your breath!

1 ABDOMINAL CRUNCH

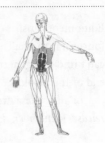

TARGET MUSCLES: Abdominals
BENEFIT: Strengthens and tones the
abdomen from sternum to pelvis,
giving a rippled appearance to the front torso.

- ○ Lie supine on the floor with knees raised
  and feet on the floor.
- ○ Place hands lightly behind the head,
  elbows out to the side.
- ○ Exhale as you contract the abs and simultaneously lift upper and
  lower torso.
- ○ Eyes should be focused toward the ceiling.

TRAINING TIPS
DO:

- ○ If you're a beginner, support the weight of the head, neck, and
  shoulders throughout the exercise with a rolled towel.
- ○ Keep the head at a natural extension from the spine to avoid neck
  strain.
- ○ Be aware if you feel tightness or pain in the muscles of the neck or
  upper back—you may be trying too hard.

DON'T:

- ○ Jerk up and drop down.
- ○ Drop the chin to the chest.
- ○ Allow the neck to move.

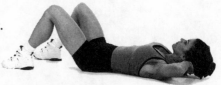

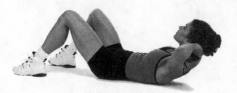

2 MODIFIED PUSH-UP

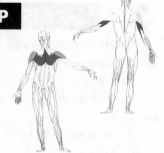

TARGET MUSCLES: Pectorals, Deltoids, Triceps

BENEFIT: Lifts breasts. Strengthens the chest, shoulders, and upper back.

- Start on your knees with your shoelaces facing the floor.
- Lean forward and support your weight with your hands, keeping them slightly more than shoulder-width apart.
- Lower your torso to one inch off the floor.
- Exhale as you push your body up until arms are extended.
- For advanced levels, lift the knees and support body weight on the toes.

TRAINING TIPS

DO:

- Use controlled movement.
- Keep your head and elbows parallel with your shoulders.
- Keep your back flat and knees flexed.

DON'T:

- Drop your head as you lower to the mat.
- Arch your back.
- Lock your elbows.

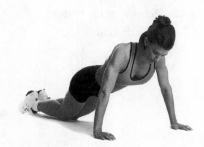

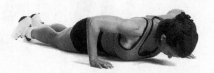

3   SQUAT

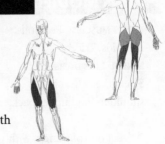

TARGET MUSCLES: Gluteals, Hamstrings, Quadriceps
BENEFIT: Shapes and strengthens the lower body like no other exercise.

- Stand with your feet shoulder-width apart.
- Lower your buttocks until just above knee level.
- Exhale as you return to standing.
- Keep your back straight and carefully control your descent.

TRAINING TIPS
DO:

- Go as low as you can without discomfort.
- Use weights if you choose (3–5 lbs. for beginners; 8–20 lbs. for advanced exercisers).

DON'T:

- Pitch the heels forward.
- Let your heels "pop" off the floor as you descend.
- "Bounce" at the bottom of the descent.

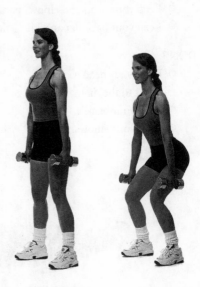

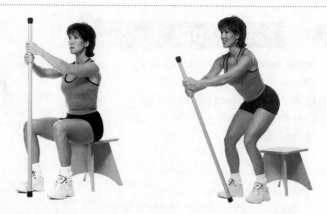

BEGINNER MODIFICATION #1:

- Use a dowel and a stool to aid in learning proper form.
- Begin seated and hold dowel vertically between the feet.
- Pressing through the heels, lift the glutes and partially stand.
- Hold briefly and return to seated position.

BEGINNER MODIFICATION #2:

- Use a dowel on a 1- or 2-inch board under the heels to help maintain an erect torso.
- Elevate your heels to allow the torso to descend easily into the gluteal training zone.

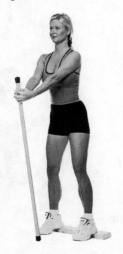
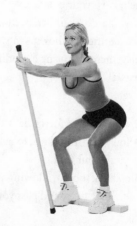

4 DIP

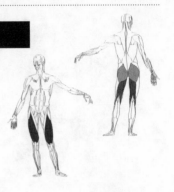

TARGET MUSCLES: Gluteals, Hamstrings, Quadriceps

BENEFIT: Strengthens hips and thighs. Provides extra toning for the bottom of the buttocks.

○ Hold a dowel outside the leg you will be moving.
○ Step back with one foot until the front thigh is almost parallel to the floor.
○ Return to starting position.
○ You will feel the muscles of the thighs and buttocks in the stationary leg.
○ Use a dumbbell (3–5 lbs. for beginners; 7–12 lbs. for advanced exercisers) to increase effectiveness.

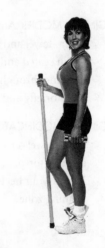

TRAINING TIPS

DO:

○ Keep the chest vertical.
○ Use a high-backed chair or dowel to help keep your balance.
○ If you are a beginner, become accustomed to the dips in small increments by using a modified, partial descent.

DON'T:

○ Pitch the torso forward.
○ Allow your front knee to extend beyond your foot.
○ Step back too far, allowing your back knee to extend past your hip.

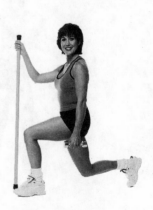

5 ROW

TARGET MUSCLES: Lattissimus Dorsi
BENEFIT: Reshapes and stretches the back.

- Stand with your feet apart.
- Use a step or the seat of a chair for support. Lean forward and place your right hand on the chair. Hold a dumbbell (3–5 lbs. for beginners; 10–25 lbs. for advanced exercisers) in your left hand.
- Keep your back parallel to the floor.
- Extend the dumbbell the full length of your arm.
- Pull the weight upward to the side of the rib cage.
- Change arms and repeat movements.

TRAINING TIPS
DO:

- Contract the back muscles around the spine as you pull to top position.
- Keep your elbows close to your body during the peak contraction.
- Slowly lower the weight back to starting position.
- Contract the abdominals to protect the lower back.

DON'T:

- Let the muscles of your arms "cheat" to assist in the move—you must feel your back muscles doing the work.
- Jerk the weight up and let it "fall down."
- Lock the supporting knee. Keep it slightly flexed.

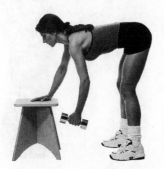 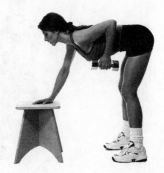

6 OVERHEAD PRESS

TARGET MUSCLES: Deltoids
BENEFIT: Strengthens and shapes the muscles on the shoulders.

- Select dumbbells (3–5 lbs. for beginners; 7–10 lbs. for advanced exercisers).
- Sit or stand with feet at shoulder-width apart.
- Contract abdominals to help stabilize torso.
- Hold dumbbells with straight wrists, palms facing forward.
- Press dumbbells straight overhead, rotating palms inward and exhaling on the lift. Return to start position slowly.

TRAINING TIPS
DO:
- Keep the weights steady when you hit the down position, stopping the weights at your ears.
- Keep the torso erect and stable.

DON'T:
- Allow the weights to fall down on your shoulders.
- Slump the shoulders.
- Lock the knees. Keep them slightly flexed.

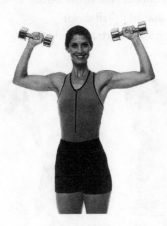
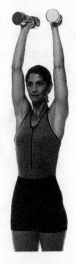

7 UPRIGHT ROW

TARGET MUSCLES: Deltoids

BENEFIT: Reshapes sloped shoulders to full shape, making the waist and hips appear smaller.

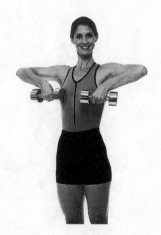

- ○ Hold 7–10 lb. dumbbells (3–5 lbs. for beginners) in front of your thighs.
- ○ Pull the weights upward, leading with your elbows as you bring the weights to shoulder level.
- ○ Exhale on the lift.
- ○ Pause briefly at the top of the move, then return to starting position.
- ○ Maintain resistance as you lower the weights.

TRAINING TIPS
DO:
- ○ Squeeze shoulder blades together at the top.
- ○ Keep a smooth rhythm to the stroke.
- ○ Keep the knees flexed.

DON'T:
- ○ Swing the weights up.
- ○ Drop the weights down.
- ○ Lead with your wrists.

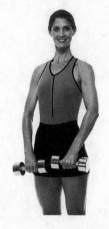

8 BICEPS CURL

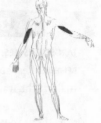

TARGET MUSCLES: Biceps

BENEFIT: Shapes and firms the front of the upper arm.

- Stand or sit on a tall box with 5–15 lb. dumbbells (3–5 lbs. for beginners) in each hand, arms extended and palms forward.
- Keeping your elbows at your waist, flex arms to lift weights to your chest.
- Pause briefly at the top of the movement, then return to starting position.
- Maintain resistance as you lower the weights.

TRAINING TIPS
DO:

- Keep the spine erect and knees unlocked.
- Lower the weights slowly.

DON'T:

- Allow the chest to slump forward.
- Curl your wrists at the top of the movement.

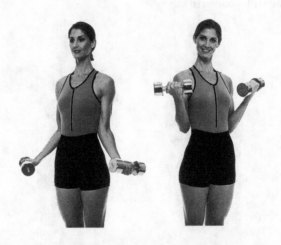

9 TRICEPS FRENCH PRESS

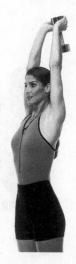

TARGET MUSCLES: Triceps

BENEFIT: Shapes and firms the back of the upper arm.

- Select one 7–10 lb. dumbbell (3–5 lbs. for beginners).
- Stand or sit on a tall box, holding dumbbell behind your head.
- Keeping your elbows close to your head, lift the weight straight up, fully extending your arms and exhaling as you lift.
- Pause briefly at the top of the movement, then return to starting position, maintaining resistance on the way down.
- Allow only the forearms to move—the upper arms should remain stationary and close to the head.

TRAINING TIPS
DO:

- Keep the elbows close to the head.
- Contract the triceps at the top of the stroke.

DON'T:

- Allow the weight to fall down into the start position.
- Allow the elbows to fan out away from the head.

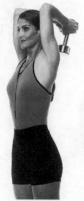

10 SEATED ROW

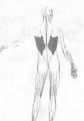

TARGET MUSCLES: Rhomboids, Latissimus Dorsi
BENEFIT: Shapes the muscles of the midback and improves posture.

○ Select two 5–10 lb. dumbbells (3–5 lbs. for beginners).
○ In a seated position, pitch the chest forward and extend the arms, with the dumbbells in each hand, palms facing inward.
○ Contract the muscle around the spine to bring your shoulder blades together.
○ Pause briefly and return to starting position, maintaining resistance as you lower the weights.

TRAINING TIPS
DO:
○ Feel the muscles of the back as you lift the weights.
○ Flex your elbows slightly.

DON'T:
○ Use the arm muscles to lift and lower the weights.

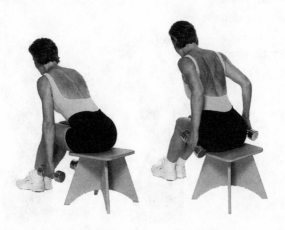

11   CALF LIFT

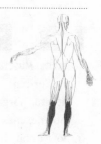

TARGET MUSCLES: Calves, Achilles' Tendon
BENEFIT: Shapes and defines the calf.

- Use a dowel, board, and step to position
  yourself for a full calf contraction.
- Allow your heel to fully stretch and extend
  down to starting position.
- As you feel your muscle contract, elevate your torso to its highest
  position.
- Briefly hold the peak contraction, then slowly return to starting
  position.

TRAINING TIPS
DO:

- Add extra resistance by holding one 5–10 lb. dumbbell on the same
  side as the working leg.
- Contract the calf muscle as you fully extend the lower leg.
- Balance your weight on the ball of your foot.

DON'T:

- Allow the heel to plunge
  to the floor on the descent.

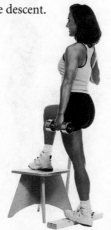
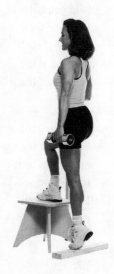

12 — LEG PRESS

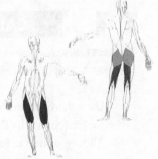

TARGET MUSCLES: Gluteals, Hamstrings, Quadriceps

BENEFIT: Targets the buttocks like no other exercise. Shapes all areas of lower body beautifully.

○ Position one foot in the center of a tall box, with your other foot close to the step and aligned directly under your hip.

○ Rise up on the ball of your "floor" foot and lift your torso up in a smooth, controlled movement, keeping chest vertical and exhaling as you lift.

○ Return to starting position with controlled movement.

○ To intensify, add dumbbells or a barbell.

TRAINING TIPS
DO:

○ Hold a dowel on the same side as your "floor" leg to help you balance.

○ Beginners may wish to keep their "floor" foot flat at the bottom of the move.

DON'T:

○ Pitch forward.

○ Bounce at the top or bottom of the movement.

○ Push off with your "floor" foot.

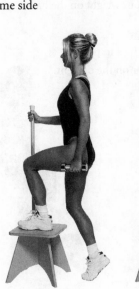

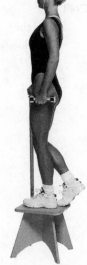

THE STRETCHES

FIRM stretches, which should be done every day, are designed to relax and elongate all the major muscles of your body. They improve the mind-body connection and allow you to feel what is happening in your body as you exercise.

Stretch Basics

These basic compulsories increase flexibility in the body and improve posture. Hold either static or with a slight pulse for about ten seconds, and try to perform the stretches after you have completed about three to four minutes of movement. As we age, we need to increase the number of minutes we spend stretching. In our twenties, we need about five to ten minutes a day. By the time we reach our fifties, we need about thirty to forty minutes each day.

All stretches can be more effective through breath control. As you stretch, practice the basic technique of contracting the internal diaphragm with breathing. Combine the inhale with an internal lift. Combine the exhale with an internal release. Do several strong contractions on each stretch. This will increase your ability to focus on the exercises and to feel the activation of each stretch. Make it a habit to include these inner compulsories every time you stretch.

In all these exercises, you should inhale and contract the diaphragm as you activate the stretch and exhale from the diaphragm as you release the stretch.

1 TRUNK LATERAL FLEXION

BENEFIT: Stretches the trunk of the body.

- ○ Hold a dowel outside the feet on one side of the body.
- ○ Lift your free arm overhead and stretch the side of the rib cage.
- ○ Intensify the stretch by lifting the shoulders away from the hip.
- ○ Move the dowel to the other side of your body and repeat.

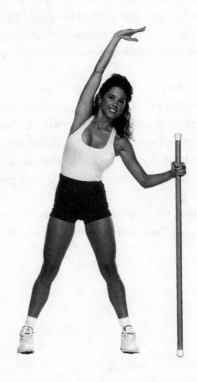

2 QUADRICEPS STRETCH

BENEFIT: Stretches the large muscle of the frontal leg, the quadriceps.

○ Hold a dowel in front of the nonstretching leg.
○ While holding the ankle (not the foot!) in your hand, flex the knee and activate the stretch with a pelvic tuck.
○ Keep your knees close together throughout the stretch.
○ Repeat with other leg.

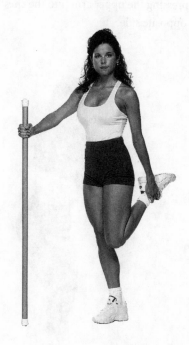

3 STANDING HAMSTRING/ DELTOID STRETCH

BENEFIT: Simultaneously stretches the back of the leg and the medial deltoid of the shoulder.

○ From a standing position, place one foot in front of the body and flex the frontal heel.

○ Flex the back knee and lean slightly forward from the hip.

○ Activate the hamstring stretch by slightly arching the lower back and lifting the gluteals.

○ Bring the arm across and into the chest to activate the shoulder stretch by pressing the upper arm into the chest.

○ Repeat on opposite side.

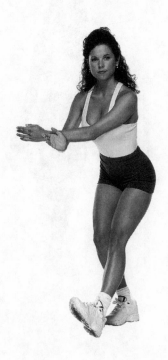

4   SPINAL ROCK

BENEFIT: Allows the lower spine to move through its entire range of motion.

- Stand with your feet hip-distance apart, toes forward.
- Keep your body weight in the heels, bend your knees, and place your hands on the thighs.
- Lower the head and drop the chin to the chest.
- Tuck the pelvis under and lift the shoulders and lower back to make a full spinal contraction.
- Release by allowing the head to come up and the entire spine to relax and arch.

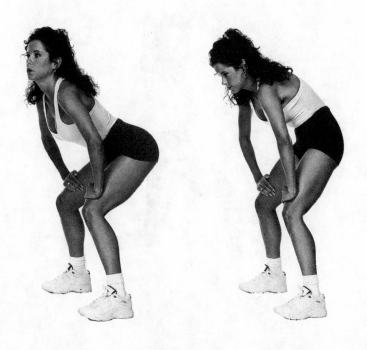

5 HIP FLEXOR/TRICEPS STRETCH

BENEFIT: Increases the range of motion in the front of the hip socket and the flexibility in the back of the arm, or triceps.

○ From an erect position, step forward with the right leg, lift the heel on the left leg, and dip down to flex the knee.
○ With both arms overhead, hold the elbow of the left arm and pull inward.
○ Repeat on opposite side.
○ Each stretch can be performed individually.

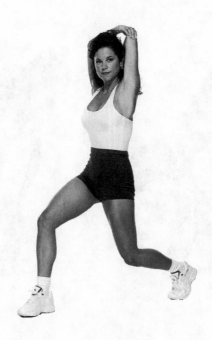

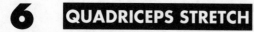

6 **QUADRICEPS STRETCH**

BENEFIT: Stretches the large muscle of the frontal leg, the quadriceps.

○ While lying on your side, flex your top knee and hold your ankle.

○ As you pull your foot to your hip, tuck your hips under to activate the stretch.

○ Repeat on opposite leg.

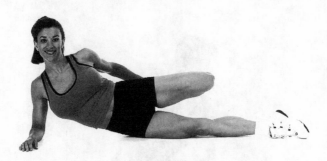

7   GROIN STRETCH

BENEFIT: Increases flexibility in the hip joints and leg adductors.

- Sit on a tall box.
- Turn toes out, with the heels directly under the knees.
- To activate the stretch, flex the torso forward.
- Keep the back flat with the chest lifted and the shoulders back.

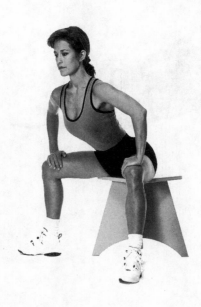

8 GROIN STRETCH WITH PELVIC CONTRACTIONS

BENEFIT: In addition to the basic groin stretch, this exercise strengthens the pelvic floor.

○ As you assume an activated groin stretch, add internal contractions with rhythmical breathing.

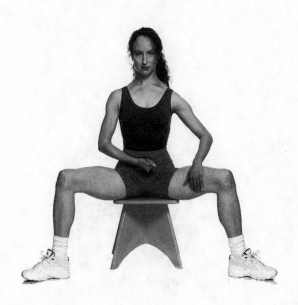

9 HIP STRETCH

BENEFIT: Increases the external rotation of the hip socket.

○ Place an ankle on the opposing thigh.
○ Keeping the back straight and the shoulders lifted, pitch slightly forward.
○ Press downward on the open knee.
○ Repeat on the opposing leg.

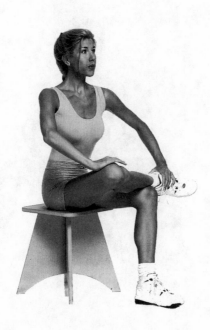

10 ▮ CAT BACK

BENEFIT: Allows the upper spine to move through its entire range of motion.

- ○ Inhale, contract the internal diaphragm, and lift the upper back as you drop the chin on the chest.
- ○ Exhale and release the internal diaphragm as you release the spine.

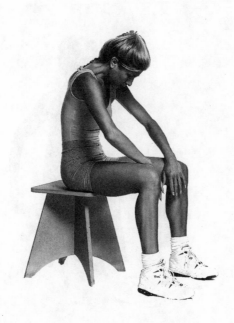

11 SWAN CHEST STRETCH

BENEFIT: Stretches the muscles of the chest and shoulders.

○ Hold the back edges of your chair or stool with both hands.
○ Use the arms to lift the face and chest upward to activate the stretch.
○ Inhaling, squeeze the shoulder blades together. Exhale and round the shoulders forward as you release.

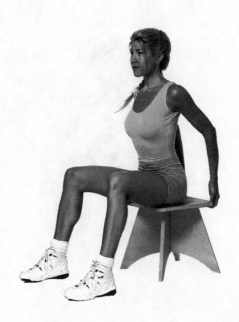

12 SEATED HAMSTRING STRETCH WITH FRONTAL SWEEP

BENEFIT: Stretches the large muscle at the back of the leg. The extended arm adds additional body weight to increase the effectiveness of the stretch.

- While seated, hold the dowel outside the extended working leg.
- Extend dowel-side leg forward, placing the heel on the floor and pointing the toes to the ceiling.
- Maintain a straight back and lean forward slightly, while lifting your free arm to the side of your head.
- Repeat on opposite side.

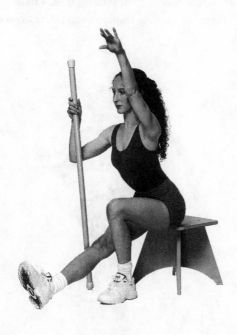

SWEAT MINUTES

Just sixty seconds of these activities will help you become accustomed to the idea of vigorous exercise and will give you short bursts of energy throughout the day. When you think it's too hard, try just a little more. You may surprise yourself. Sweat Minutes won't burn fat or train your heart, but they're excellent practice for the real thing!

1   MARCHES

The simplest of all aerobic movements, this step can be performed in time to your favorite up-tempo tune.

- Move the opposing arm and leg on each stroke.
- March up, not down.
- Make sure the entire foot strikes the floor each time.
- Pump the arms by moving from the shoulders to increase aerobic intensity.

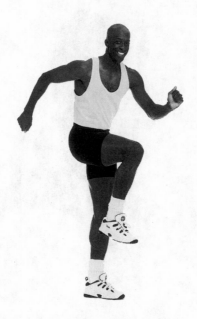

2 KICKS

Kicks are a fabulous toner for the upper thighs and buttocks.

○ From a standing position, pull your leg up and out by bringing your knee into your torso.
○ Kick the working leg by extending the knee joint and directing the heel toward an imaginary target.
○ Hold both arms into the chest and allow the torso to lean over and down in the opposite direction from the kicking leg.
○ For additional aerobic benefit, add an arm punch with the kick, using the arm on the same side of the body.

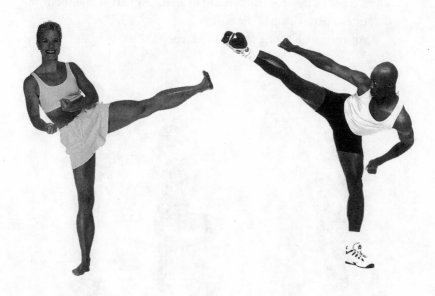

3 TALL BOX CLIMB

A famous FIRM invention and a favorite of all instructors and clients in our studios. Not only does it tone the buttocks and thighs, it burns fat! In our classes, we do just enough of this cardio pumper to keep the heart rate high between sets of weight exercises.

- ○ Stand directly behind the box, feet together and hands on hips. Keep your head up and eyes on the box.
- ○ Place right foot in center of step.
- ○ Lift body and bring left foot up to the top.
- ○ Step down with the right leg, follow with left leg, and repeat movement.
- ○ Do not let the chest fall forward or allow any part of your body to extend past the top of the box.
- ○ Alternate with left leg forward and repeat.

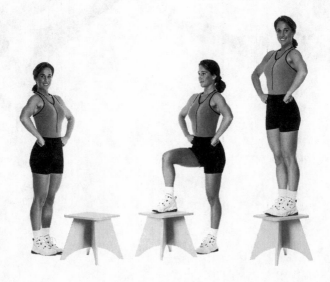

4 PLYOMETRICS

This is another favorite intensifier used during our FIRM classes. Short sets of jumps can get your heart rate up quickly.

- Jump out one time.
- Jump in two times.
- Vary the pace with some low jumps and some high jumps.
- Use the arms to power up on each jump.
- Descend into a slight squat at the bottom of each jump, with arms thrust forward.

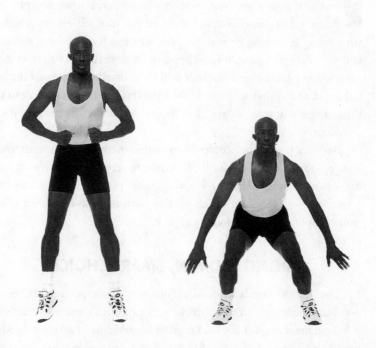

CHAPTER 6

FIRM
spirits

Exercise is a great awakener. Not only do you experience new physical strength and shapeliness; you also find that your self-esteem is higher, your energy level is far more dynamic, your stress level has been reduced, and your dreams and ambitions begin to become reality. You started by consciously establishing a workout goal for yourself. You got past the initial dread and embarrassment to the exhilaration, and you began to see the changes you were looking for. You're physically stronger and more confident.

But what you've also acquired is mental strength and inner confidence. Now you are able, perhaps for the first time, to set goals in all areas of your life. You have awakened to the workout's larger purpose: It is a foundation for a richer existence, in which you, as a strong, self-actualized FIRM woman, opt for what you want, and get it!

STRONG WOMEN, SMART CHOICES

The FIRM woman is focused, but not obsessive; competitive with herself, not with others; strong, but not offensive; tough when the situation calls for it, but not mean or cruel. She has her priorities straight, and acknowledges her limitations. Her life is rich and full, but does not overwhelm her. She never stops learning and never stops setting new goals. She doesn't try to conform to the stereotypical media ideal of beautiful and sexy, nor to the feminist notion that a woman must be perfect at everything she does. She has endured the often painful process of change, and it has given her the courage to lead.

In our own family, there is a tradition of strong women playing leadership roles that goes back several generations. Our mother, as we've said, was a freethinker, who put the needs of her family above convention. Both our maternal grandmother, Beatrice Spearman Stanley, and paternal grandmother, Ruth Montgomery Benson, taught school. Beatrice Spearman Stanley became a principal and later went on to teach herself architecture and become a successful real estate developer.

Our maternal great-grandmother, Mary Stanley Hillegas, known as "the Belle of Columbia," ran a boardinghouse during Reconstruction years, when family finances were devastated by the Civil War. And a great-great-aunt was the first superintendent of schools in the city.

These were women who were not afraid of hard work, and who served well the family, the community, and the workplace. They were entrepreneurs of a sort, remarkable for their eras, and positive role models for us. We have to wonder if we would be writing this book if it weren't for them.

Although we knew our matriarchs sacrificed to achieve their goals, it wasn't until we actually had to put our own project together that we truly understood what that meant. Sheer mental strength and focusing on the goal allowed us to succeed and gave us the confidence to tackle other projects. Whatever you call it—self-discipline, desire, mental strength—it's something valuable to us all.

DEAR FIRM

"Because of The FIRM I now make healthful choices in all aspects of my life— diet, activities, vacation."

ELIZABETH H., 37,
registered nurse

BABE-ISM VS. FIRM-ISM

Although the fitness business frequently is perceived as being driven by hardbodies, babes, or hunks, the secondary benefits of physical strength are invaluable to us all. Thomas Jefferson wrote, "A strong body makes the mind strong." And we at The FIRM acknowledge that mental strength is key to personal happiness.

FIRM clients and instructors know that physical strength increases mental strength—and self-esteem. As self-esteem increases, so does self-confidence. And self-confidence increases our ability to achieve our goals and to experience life to the fullest.

The FIRM teaches that by maintaining strong mental and physical strength (and corresponding benefits) we become secure in our own being and our own talents and gifts. We can afford to be magnanimous, to acknowledge others' contributions or assets without envy. We can accept constructive criticism without defensiveness and realize that such comments may actually improve our performance. We know that traditional female competitiveness, usually shown in forms such as gossip, sarcasm, or backbiting, comes from insecure individuals with low self-esteem.

The FIRM acknowledges that some personality types are more competitive than others. When we release inner anger and frustration through focused physical activities, we gain positive physical energy that then can be released in healthy forms of competition. FIRM women are secure in their self-worth and are able to enjoy healthy competition.

As for the media's "babe" worship, it's important to remember that beautiful and sexy has its downside. In fact, one of the pitfalls of being a babe or a hunk is that narcissism can sometimes prevent a person from developing significant intimate relations with other people. These media darlings have to fight harder to develop their humanity because of the lure and seductiveness of narcissism.

At The FIRM, we feel it's our responsibility, in many ways, to lead women into alternatives to the babe model. We encourage an enjoyment of other aspects of being female, such as confidence, grace, youthful energy, style, decisiveness, and sensuality. And we promote the concept that a toned body combined with a sharp mind is a seductive and alluring package.

The mind is a great facilitator, which you must strengthen just as you strengthen a muscle. Educating oneself takes time and effort, but it's a wonderful gift to give yourself, still vibrant when beauty has faded. If we had to choose between being beautiful and never sweating, on the one hand, or being ordinary and able to handle ourselves in a variety of situations, on the other hand, we'd choose "ordinary" without a second thought!

"The FIRM has changed my life in so many ways. I honestly feel that I don't get sick as often, due to being stronger. I suffer from PMS and The FIRM has helped me tremendously with the stress and irritability that come with it. It has helped me with my self-esteem. I feel all-over happier with my life because of The FIRM."

TRACEY GRAY, 32

PRACTICE THE CLASSICAL IDEAL

You really can't focus on exercise and diet without considering who you are and how you relate to others. Once you begin feeling healthy, you'll naturally begin to improve the general quality of your life. In this chapter, we'll show you how to awaken your mind to match your awakened body, and we'll give you fabulous tips for communicating the new you to others—in areas such as grooming, manners, goal-setting, and developing a sense of style. This is advice that works. Much of it has come from our personal experiences, and much more from students, instructors, and FIRM Believers.

Throughout, we urge you to keep in mind the twofold classical ideal of a Greek education, which is a perfect harmony of literary and artistic development of the mind and systematic gymnastic training of the body. Each nourishes the other; the mind nurtures the body, and the body supports full mental flowering.

Seek your own sense of peace amid the chaos of living.

Strive for balance, symmetry, and happiness in all things.

Remember that knowledge is power, and that true beauty comes from within.

It is only through continuous learning every day of your life that you direct your existence in a positive way.

And never forget that gentleness and strength are not in opposition but in confluence.

"I hate to sound like I am gushing, but The FIRM is the most incredible inspiration to shape up I've ever used, and I've tried everything. My butt is completely resculpted! Can I tell you I have no cellulite anymore? I mean it's gone!"

CHRISTINE T., 24,
securities paralegal

ANIMAL INSTINCTS

One of the things that has always intrigued us is why humans are never motivated to get in shape unless they're in a period of active change—whether pleasant or catastrophic. For instance, courtship falls in the very pleasant realm, and the death of a spouse in the catastrophic. But it's usually under those circumstances that people display the same reliance on the physical and external, on our animal nature, if you will.

There are so many ways we can suppress that animal nature. It's only when we're elated or devastated or threatened with poor health that we look at ourselves physically. That's unfortunate because human beings really are happiest when we fulfill all aspects of our humanity.

"I have maintained a sixty-seven-pound weight loss for eight years thanks to The FIRM. I have been able to reshape my body; therefore I have gained the confidence to reshape my life."

HIAM BRINGIKJI, 33,
real estate agent, West Bloomfield, Michigan

MASTERING THE ANIMAL DIMENSION

If you've led a sedentary life, you could think of yourself as an animal imprisoned in the cage of metropolitan, civilized living. Your personality and basic nature are affected by this. Our animal nature is constantly subdued by the demands of civilization. Only in a few things, such as sex, manual labor, exercise or sports, can our bodies function as they were meant to—as perfectly designed machines created for hard work. And yet we spend all our lives trying to exert mastery over our animal dimension. When we're growing up, we often don't have control of our emotions, and we must invest considerable energy in learning how to curb our impulses.

One of the actions many women take when they start an exercise program is to set internal goals for themselves, possibly for the first time in their lives. Until then, they've allowed others—parents, teachers, bosses, boyfriends, husbands—to set goals for them. Frequently one of the first goals is mastery of personal energy. People are, by nature, lazy, and all of us have the irrefutable desire for a quick fix and immediate satisfaction. It's hard to fight inertia, just as it's hard to set your own goals.

Exercise is one of the few areas of people's lives—perhaps in women's lives particularly—where they *can* set concrete goals and actualize them!

Setting goals is what seems to us so unique about exercise: You set a goal and get something you can measure. You can actually see something happening, something changing. What this does is boost self-esteem because nothing makes you feel more empowered than achieving a goal. In fact, your self-confidence rises in direct proportion to your ability to actualize goals.

DEAR FIRM

"Yesterday, at a party, my husband said I was the best-looking and most fit woman there! I was also one of the oldest women there!!! My husband also said my thighs looked great in jeans and that I had the greatest behind. I was fat and turning thirty-five. Now I'll be forty and look great."

**VICKI MAYER, 39,
childbirth educator, Everett, Washington**

FIRM GROOMING

Although The FIRM teaches women that strength of body and mind are true beauty, we can't deny that we are visual creatures and that presentation does matter. We know this from grooming instructors and video leads. (While these women are talented and strong leaders in their own right, video training demands a new level of performance.)

Grooming is another key to confidence. It shows respect for the self and for others. Still, many people disregard it. If they're beautiful, they don't think it's important. If they're average, they think it's not going to help. Are they ever wrong!

Tasteful grooming is a subtle yet powerful communicator. And, having seen the world through the camera lens, we know that little things matter. We believe you should know how you look from the back, practice good diction and grammar, and be aware of body language. You should learn to take care of your skin and maintain manicured hands and feet. Remember that a purse isn't a tote bag or a trash receptacle. Cleanliness and neatness do matter.

Our ultimate goal should be to have no limits on our ability to achieve our dreams. It's only too easy to relax and appear unkempt. The trick is to practice certain self-disciplines at all times so that the good habits become second nature to us. We can be comfortable whether dining with the president of a large company, visiting a close friend's grandmother, or presenting new ideas to business associates.

Remember that refinement in detail or extremities indicates a high level of discipline and development. For the ballet dancer, this is controlled hands and feet even when executing highly physical movements. For the musician, this is complete control over even the small ornamental embellishments. In FIRM grooming, this refinement encompasses personal grooming, physical presentation, and intellectual activity.

Nonverbal communication is useful to everyone. As we go through life, people form quick and vivid impressions of us. With attention to our physical presentation we can enhance our ability to communicate with others through our unique style and to create a more satisfying life for ourselves.

"My sex life is so much better. Being in shape makes you feel so much sexier."

TRICIA JONES, 32,
homemaker, Kingsburg, California

INVENTING YOUR ATHLETIC STYLE

Workouts, quite frankly, are a time to sweat and be an animal. As you begin to become more fit and confident, choose loose-fitting, brief clothes that reveal working muscles. Keep your arms and legs bare so that you'll be able to see each muscle as it works. Not only can you watch the muscle and make sure your form is correct, but nothing is quite as inspiring as seeing changes in your muscular development. A major aspect of developing and toning individual muscles is mental focus. By watching the muscle as you're working it, you enhance your concentration, which produces faster results.

As your figure changes, you'll want to adjust your athletic wardrobe. For one thing, you'll sweat more, so your clothes will have to be layered to accommodate the changes in your body temperature. This way you can dress for a workout and gradually peel off layers as you become hotter. To prevent becoming chilled, you simply reverse the process. Many exercisers need to see the working muscle in a mirror to stay motivated. This is not about vanity; it's about body alignment, form, breathing, technique, focusing, and getting through the set.

Keep your hair off your face—in a ponytail, barrettes, or a sweatband—so you won't inhibit your ability to sweat, move, and focus. Exercise is the one life situation where it's a plus to get down and sweaty!

"The FIRM gave me something to strive for, by seeing the muscular definition of the instructors and believing I could do that, too."

HEATHER SAPIRO, 40,
pet nanny, Wheaton, Illinois

DEVELOPING YOUR BEST LOOK

Style is as timeless as it is individual. Fashions may change each year, but true style, which is yours and yours alone, never grows dated. With your new body and mindset, you'll be ready to make your wardrobe a personal signature. But even when you're still on the road to your fitness goal, you should start creatively attacking your image.

It's hard to believe, but many women have never analyzed their bodies in front of a full-length mirror—an imperative step to deciding which body parts you want to highlight and which you want to play down. Always consider the importance of optical illusion when choosing how you dress:

- Is your body pear-shaped? Consider light colors above the waist and dark colors below, while you reduce body fat and use heavy weights for your upper body.
- Do you have thick ankles and knees? You *can't* change your joint size—it's part of your genetic blueprint—but you *can* make pants a wardrobe staple. As you reduce body fat, make sure the pants you choose accent your buttocks and waist, and make up for what you conceal by showing off more perfect areas.
- Is your tummy round or full? Make extensive use of the food diary: You could have a food allergy that is causing you to bloat. As you continue reducing body fat and concentrating on abdominal training, wear loose-fitting, dark tops.
- Do you have beautiful breasts and/or a great back? Select styles to accentuate your best features: Low-cut, or the virtually backless, dresses so popular today showcase hard-earned muscle, and scoop necklines display pectorals and breasts.
- Are your arms your best body part? Be sure to keep your fat layer low enough to reveal upper body definition, then plan your wardrobe for a year-round display of muscle. Sleeveless tops can be layered with a vest, cardigan, coat, or jacket.

Above all, don't be afraid to show off your assets!

BASIC NEUTRALS: THE KEY TO STUNNING

When you're improving your image with a new approach, construct your wardrobe in monochromatic silhouettes: black first, then other neutrals. You can add more dramatic color once you've identified your best shapes and looks.

A hint about wearing dark colors: You'll want to use a lint brush every time you get dressed (whether or not you have a pet that sheds), and never forget to pack one in your car and on your travels.

Once you've established your personal best weight and mastered the elements of styles and cuts in basic black, try venturing into gray, beige, and other muted neutrals. Light-colored neutrals, especially small accents of pink, are particularly flattering next to the face.

All shoes, belts, and handbags should also be in black. Select jewelry either in gold or silver, but not both unless it's in your budget.

Unless you have the perfect body and plenty of money, your detail, texture, and pattern should be limited to scarves and jewelry. Prints, if used at all, should be small-scale and neutral. Except for the rare accent piece, place your wardrobe dollars elsewhere—on high-quality shoes, belts, purses, etc.

Until you become the you that you always wanted to be, keep everything simple and remember that less is more. Generally, a monochromatic look of one color from head to foot is most striking and effective. Accent with colorful scarves and unusual jewelry. Self-adornment is a very basic human expression; do it with savvy.

And a quick word about underwear (something people don't usually think about.) During the cold months, underwear basics should be black and *in perfect condition*. When necessary, beige and white can be introduced in the summer under lighter colored garments. Keep your rear views perfect! Clip and removal labels from garments. You may enjoy trying thongs, which are underpants that leave the buttocks uncovered and have no panty lines. Nothing looks better than firm gluteals; and nothing looks worse that visible panty lines interrupting smooth, toned buttocks.

Always examine bras before purchasing them. Don't fall for wild colors or patterns; look instead for good construction and quality lace.

"After my husband left me for a younger woman, I felt miserable about myself. Since using The FIRM, I feel attractive again, and I have a wonderful new beau."

JULIE ANNE RODAK, 32,
attorney, Slingerlands, New York

PERSONAL GROOMING

Increased physical fitness and confidence lead to a change in dressing patterns. In order to be totally comfortable during exercise, groom your body for total freedom of movement. Your skin and hair are highly visible and create a moving, tangible aura as you sweat.

The intricacies of hygiene are as old as civilization itself. The Egyptians maintained high standards of cleanliness. The Greeks exercised in the nude so that, during public competitions, artists were able to study carefully the human physique. Through their representations of those bodies, civilization was introduced to beautiful and realistic sculpture. Through aqueducts, the Romans had plenty of fresh water for public baths. In the ancient world, cleanliness was a natural expression of good health.

However, after the fall of the Roman Empire, Europe was plunged into the savage one thousand years called the Dark Ages, a period that saw the rise of hideous diseases, such as the Black Death. During the sixteenth and seventeenth centuries, Europeans—probably because of water-borne viruses such as typhus and cholera—developed a paranoid dread of water and considered the act of bathing dangerous. Public baths were banned out of fear of social and moral depravity. To counteract body odor and physical grime, the upper classes developed elaborate techniques of powdering and scenting.

Modern hygiene, in fact, is a mere 250 years old. It began when elaborate bathrooms, almost always used prior to amorous encounters, were, in the 1740s, slowly reintroduced by European aristocrats. Even today, the art of personal hygiene continues to evolve as women assert more control over their bodies.

Hair

Invest in a good haircut. Find a talented stylist who will analyze your facial proportions and design a low-maintenance athletic look just for you! Maintain the look with regular cut sessions. Select hair color with care. And if you've got them, cover your gray hairs!

Makeup

The biggest difference in updating makeup can often be made with (1) the best professional brushes and application tools and (2) colors that are right for your style and skin tone. These do not have to be high-ticket items. Artist supply stores stock good face brushes; discount stores and professional makeup supply houses stock a wide range of colors and products. Whatever you do, don't be fooled by fancy packaging. Instead, be aware of your own best colors as you incorporate new trends. It's even a good idea to take samples from your makeup collection when you shop.

Doing your face is an exercise in optical illusion, and it takes practice. The best advice usually comes from a professional makeup artist. Most important, be sure you have the professional do a face map, on which the artist will chart the best colors for your face. Take it with you when you shop. Even though you think you'll remember the colors used during a makeover, once you wash your face, you won't. So keep that record!

For exercise and sports, waterproof mascara is a must. Always carry cotton pads and a non-oily eye makeup remover solvent, like Clinique's Rinse-Off Eye Makeup Solvent, for quick touch-ups after you sweat. Elizabeth Arden Lip Fix is wonderful for keeping lipstick from bleeding outside the lip line.

Tanning Bare Limbs

As you begin to strengthen muscle and lose fat, you'll be able to wear more revealing clothing. Women with fair skin may want to consider sunless tanning lotion, which can greatly enhance the look of bare limbs, thighs, and buttocks. Believe it or not, when such lotions are skillfully applied, they look great and are faster (and *much* healthier) than sun exposure or tanning beds.

If you choose to be year-round pale, know that, because of the dangers of exposure to the sun, your look is increasingly popular and very Victorian, with lots of romantic possibilities. Whether or not you tan, never leave the house without sunscreen covering exposed areas of your body and without moisturizer (at least fifteen sun protection factor) on your face! Also, the thin skin on the sternum (breastbone) can sustain permanent sun damage in the form of leathery skin and dark freckles. Protect this area from the sun as carefully as you do your face.

Hands and Feet

The new, stylish, short, and athletic fingernails for women are wonderful time savers. All you need to do is cut them straight across and file the corners. Clean nails daily with a nail brush, soap, and cuticle pusher. Invest in the best nail tools. Tweezerman products are top of the line.

You should prepare your nails for the day just as you do your face. Experiment with a white pencil under the tips (the so-called French manicure), cuticle trimming, and oil brushing. Clear polish will give your nails a professional, manicured look. Incidentally, a truly thoughtful gesture is to do the nails of a close friend. Be sure both fingernails and toenails are manicured 365 days a year!

Beautiful Skin

The single most indispensable beauty product for your skin is sunscreen (see section above on tanning bare limbs). This becomes increasingly important as you spend more time outdoors in warm weather and—since your exercise results are making you stronger and more positively competitive—participate in outdoor sports.

Exfoliation renews and beautifies the skin. Use lubricant, soap, or glycolic acid with a natural bristle nail brush to scrub your entire body in the shower. It will remove dead skin and leave you glowing and rejuvenated from head to toe.

Schedule an occasional bath, sauna, or whirlpool immediately following your workout; they do wonders for tired muscles. Be sure to wear a deep pore cleanser as you sweat. Follow with a tightening mask. This can be used immediately after heat therapy to close pores.

Many women use Retin-A or its skin-friendly cousin Renova, relatively new products available only by prescription that erase skin lines and remove surface wrinkles and light spots.

"The FIRM makes me feel good about myself, increasing self-esteem. I feel proud of my accomplishments (body changes). I like my body better and that carries over into my sex life."

LISA OWENS, 35,
Garrison, Texas

INTIMATE GROOMING: FOR WOMEN ONLY

Happily, the female body is a pleasant and delightful mystery to men. Many American women, however, are subjected to cultural prejudices which keep us from knowing how our own bodies function. When teaching classes, we noticed that many women appeared to be completely out-of-touch with their bodies from the waist to the knees. By educating ourselves, we can add to the pleasure for our mates and maintain our personal health.

Workouts enhance the sexual experience in many ways. They make you aware of your body in a scintillating new way. Because of the freedom of athletic participation, athletic women exude a powerful physical force. Regular workouts change the way you smell. With the regular purifying effects of sweaty, vigorous exercise, the body assumes an undertone of fresh muskiness.

Strengthening your most intimate muscles with the pelvic floor exercises will increase sexual pleasure for both you and your partner. These pelvic floor muscles form a bowl, covering the bottom opening of the pelvis. Because these muscles surround the rim of the vagina (as well as its interior walls), strengthening them gives a tighter fit and permits voluntary squeezes during intimacy, so always incorporate pelvic diaphragm contractions into your workout.

Combined with her newfound flexibility, endurance, and strength, the FIRM woman can participate actively in more satisfying lovemaking, combining a variety of pelvic moves (from sensuous wavelike motions and isolated staccato movements) with pelvic contractions. You and your man will love it!

THE PELVIC FLOOR

Target muscles: Pelvic Diaphragm (or "Floor")

Benefit: Strengthens the muscles around the walls of the vagina to heighten sexual pleasure for both partners. Prevents and/or remedies urinary incontinence; eases childbirth.

○ Lie supine, knees flexed, feet flat.

○ Place one hand on the floor and rest the other gently on the abdomen.

○ Contract and internally lift the region between your genitals and anus, squeezing the muscles inward to the center of the body.

○ Results are enhanced by breath control: Inhale with the contraction and exhale during a controlled release.

○ For increased strength, vary the tempo of contractions. Variations include "the elevator," a deep sustained contraction that rises in the body; and "flutters," a series of rapid, intense, surface contractions.

○ Complete a minimum of 200 repetitions a day.

Safe, committed lovemaking is one of the great joys of life, and your genitals are worthy of great care and attention. Help what is naturally beautiful by perfecting your intimate grooming.

Waxing

A Los Angeles actress who came to South Carolina to do a movie panicked because she thought nobody outside of the big cities offered such intimate personal services as bikini waxing. We were able to assure her that bikini waxing was available throughout the country, even in Charleston and Columbia, South Carolina.

Body hair continues to be an interesting, and sometimes political, issue. It's quite all right with us if women choose not to shave their legs or armpits. For those of us who do groom these areas, we have a couple of tips. Waxing and/or electrolysis is a worthwhile luxury for removing unwanted hair for up to one month or longer. Usually applied to the legs, these techniques are also appropriate for stubborn bikini lines. (When you are at the swimming pool or wearing shorts, check to ensure you are not inadvertently showing something you'd rather keep private.) To eliminate ingrown hairs, use a nail brush or coconut loufah on the area.

Vaginal Health

The vagina continues to be a mysterious organ—unfortunately, sometimes even for women. Women should be knowledgeable about vaginal health and care.

When healthy, the vagina is a self-cleansing organ, which does not need the regular douching espoused by television advertisers. Some sources believe douching may actually promote infections. If you want to clean the vagina's natural secretions, insert clean fingers and water only. (No washcloths or soap internally.) Bidets are a wonderful tool for maintaining freshness and for quick cleaning.

Yeast infections are the results of a change in vaginal health wherein a fungus *(candida albicans)* overgrows and infects the vagina. Candida is part of the body's normal flora; thus, almost every woman will have a yeast infection at some time in her life. Yeast infections can be caused by oral contraceptives, IUDs, sexual partners, pregnancy, antibiotics, allergies, improper hygiene, consumption of refined carbohydrates and/or sugar, nutritional deficiencies and/or stress.

Much is being written about the neglect of women's health in the quest for corporate profit. For example, if an antibiotic causes a yeast infection, we shouldn't have to purchase a second antibiotic when an effective and inexpensive home remedy is available from our local drugstore. Try the remedy proven 98 percent effective in a Cornell University study. At the slightest hint of a yeast infection, insert two large gelatin capsules packed with boric acid powder (not crystals). Continue for two to three days, or as long as necessary. Make necessary lifestyle or dietary changes immediately!

STACEY MILLNER-COLLINS

AGE: 32
PROFESSION: WORKS WITH CHILDREN
WHO HAVE DEFICIT DISORDERS AND DRUG PROBLEMS

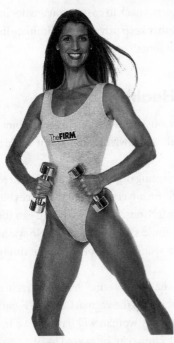

A graceful, appealing woman who radiates quiet self-assurance, Stacey came to The FIRM seven years ago after the birth of her first child. She's now the mother of two and a FIRM instructor.

Stacey is quite outspoken about her past problems. "I was the product of an upper-middle-class home," she explains, "expecting a perfection that led me into eating disorders, and I have taken myself out, pulled myself up by the bootstraps."

Stacey credits working out with causing noneating-disorder life changes. "I'm confident," she smiles. "At first it was just a purely physical change that I noticed—I had lost weight, I had gotten thinner—but this led to a generally more confident state."

This newfound physical, spiritual, and mental strength has allowed Stacey to indulge her spirit of adventure: Last year she went backpacking in Asia by herself. Her work with troubled kids entails taking them to the woods for a week at a time. And she chose to have her second baby at home, with a midwife.

Being an instructor has also helped empower her. "It takes a lot to get in front of thirty or forty people," she admits, "I mean, overcoming that fear—the number one fear of most people—of getting up in front of a crowd."

Asked what great lesson she's learned at The FIRM, Stacey replies, "The key to life is balance."

(continued)

STACEY'S TIPS FOR BEGINNERS:
- Do something you enjoy.
- Don't force yourself to do a workout you don't find fun, because you won't stay with it.
- You can exercise all you want, but it won't work if you don't maintain a healthy, moderate lifestyle.
- It's essential to combine exercise with a good diet.
- Strive for perfection, but don't expect miracles. And don't ever compare yourself to gorgeous movie stars or supermodels. Through good form and good focus, positive change will come—in as little as ten sessions!

DEVELOP IN ALL AREAS
OF YOUR LIFE

Good health and a toned, fit body free you to lead an active, productive life. You'll have the energy to socialize with people in the places that bring you pleasure. You'll find courage to develop new skills. Attaining your workout goals and enhancing your ability to focus will lead you to create an agenda for improving yourself in every area of your life.

Set regular dates to take a personal inventory of your life. Make notes (where only you can seen them) about the things in your life that you're happy about and where you want to make changes. List the reasons why you want to change. List the items in order of priority. What do you want to change more than anything else? How will you achieve those changes?

Whether it's "I want to lose three inches from my waist" or "I want to go back to school to get my degree," your goals must be realistic in order to be achieved and to build character. As you identify and refine your goals you are in many ways defining your values. Study them often to keep yourself focused. Don't try to change every aspect of your life at the same time; that's simply overwhelming for anyone. And, perhaps most important of all, learn to forgive yourself for what you see as your shortcomings. That's where awkwardness and negative self-consciousness come in. If you can get rid of your mind problems, you can perceive the world gracefully and make great strides.

Remember, top executives are encouraged to write down the exact steps necessary to achieve their business goals; why should we be any different? Seeing your goals in writing and making yourself write down the exact steps to achieve them reinforces your intentions.

DEAR FIRM

"I've spent months doing Smith/Fonda tapes with little satisfaction and insignificant results. I see the difference The FIRM has made to my body and my mind. Others see the results and comment on my muscular, firm arms, legs, etc. It's a grand cycle: I look good—I feel good—I exercise—I look good—I feel good—I exercise."

TRACIE JOHNSON SWEENEY, 38,
public relations, Narragansett, Rhode Island

THE NATURE OF DISCIPLINE

It's easy to be disciplined with things we like to do. The struggle occurs when we are confronted with boredom, disinterest, or laziness. That's when we need blind faith in future rewards. Delayed gratification takes practice. With constant exercise, that's not always easy. Anna has found that conventional forms of discipline, such as playing tennis on a regular basis, help her stay in focus. However, all individuals must find solutions that give them satisfaction and allow them to control their urges for unhealthy and nonproductive activity. Here again, it's a question of focusing and building on goals, and enlarging what it means to achieve goals in every area of your existence. Aristotle was right when he observed that habits eventually turn into lifestyles.

Self-discipline can become a philosophy of life. As we discipline ourselves in one way, we find it easier to discipline ourselves in other ways. Self-discipline allows us to achieve our goals, to have more control over our own lives. Self-discipline eventually becomes a painless habit.

Frequently, the greatest satisfaction comes from doing what you think is the most difficult, the most horrible, the most torturous—whether it be Cynthia's cold calls, the toughest workout you've ever attempted, or apologizing to a loved one whose feelings you've deeply hurt. It's not easy to tackle these challenges. We see it in exercise as we see it in life. It's called workout dread.

Workout dread initially sets in when you've established a new goal; if you stick with it, exhilaration eventually follows. Converting dread into exhilaration requires discipline, and the only thing that gets you through is your inner core of values. However, sticking with it until you feel the exhilaration is about training to be a champion.

There are many, many things you can do to help yourself focus and persevere. You must discover what they are just as you must reach inside yourself to find out who you really are and what makes you unique.

We all want to live life to the hilt. When you challenge yourself you experience true exhilaration. Here are some suggestions for extending your newfound confidence out into the world.

CULTIVATE GOOD MANNERS

Manners are what separate us from primitive societies; they're a highly evolved code of behavior that makes society harmonious and pleasant. Manners facilitate life and are designed to make others comfortable. In contrast to many hard-edged gyms, we strive to make sure that all instructors and clients of The FIRM behave with kindness and consideration toward everyone, no matter what their ranking in the fitness hierarchy. We also encourage thinking that says that the small courtesies make life more pleasant, and we strongly believe that everything pleasant in our daily existence is good for us. This extends beyond the gym into normal social intercourse.

Our present day society may seem less than civil, but there are rules. To bone up, read etiquette books, both old and new (there have been a spate of them published recently). Remember, there are two things that people will never tell you but will always hold against you. One is bad grammar, the other is bad manners. Only supermodels or movie stars can get away with such unattractive habits as chewing gum in public, chewing food with their mouths open, or fiddling with their faces or hair in public. We find that everyone believes that they don't do these things, but don't take chances; check to see if you might be guilty. (Even a famous pop music star turned actress was rumored to have hired a manners coach.) Once, when an instructor trainee was chewing gum in the FIRM studio, we asked if she knew not to chew gum in public; the instructor said she had never heard of this. A nearby client who worked for an employment agency for the legal profession spoke up and said that if a job applicant showed up chewing gum, he or she was automatically disqualified!

Sending thank-you notes is an old but lovely tradition that we are glad to see is coming back in style. Writing a note at the right time is not only thoughtful, but it can also facilitate social situations. Improve your penmanship; elegant, legible handwriting is always a treasure. And with the new technological advances, you can fax or e-mail a thank-you message and have it received immediately.

Manners are the grace of the spirit. As your body becomes firmer and more lithe, so should your consideration of others. Social ease and physical ease are meant to fuse in the classical fashion, with one nourishing the other. Not only will you feel more comfortable in a social situation, but others will find you a delight to be around.

DEAR FIRM

"I look forward to exercise because after I work out with weights I feel like I could conquer the world. It makes me rethink my feelings on being thin or skinny. The FIRM has made me so strong, it will probably add years to my life, because I'm doing something good for my body."

LESIA SWINT, 27,
Statesboro, Georgia

REFINE YOUR PHYSICAL GRACE
AND MOVEMENT

There are many ways to enhance grace and movement, but your ideal should be combining confidence with grace. During our FIRM instructor training program, practice workout tapes are made of each new teacher.

CAROL BRITTON MILLER

AGE: 40   PROFESSION: RETAIL CLOTHING REPRESENTATIVE

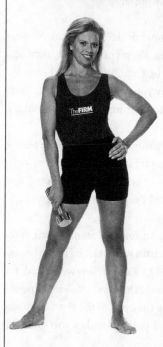

This chic, svelte blonde has been teaching at The FIRM since 1983. She became an instructor when one of The FIRM managers told her she needed a challenge. During her years working out, that need for challenge has served her well in some rough times.

"I got a divorce," she explains. "I've gotten remarried. I have step-children. As far as working out goes, the nicest thing to me is that, in instructing, we change the routines often so the session never gets stale, never gets old."

Carol travels a lot for business and, when she's on the road, takes classes. "All the time," she says, "I'm seeing stuff being introduced in the larger cities that we've been doing for a year. But it's just because of Anna's foresight. It's almost as if she's an exercise fortune teller."

When asked if FIRM thinking helped her make a better marital choice the second time, Carol replies, "I was married to my first husband for eighteen months, and all the time, he was having an affair. After that, I went for three or four years and just saw no one. I worked out. I mean, it was my life. Then, when I started dating again, I needed the self-boosting. And the support system. Some people go to church. Some people go to AA. I came here. My present husband and I have been happily married for two years. I've been around for a long time, but I've got to tell you, exercise helps my sanity!"

CAROL'S TIPS FOR BEGINNERS:

○ Strong bodies create strong minds, and keep you from making the same mistakes twice.

○ Like The FIRM program itself, you must keep innovating and setting new goals—you'll be surprised how far you can stretch.

○ Luck is about the body you were born with; work is about the body you vow to have.

The revelation of invisible habits in both voice and movement is perhaps the most valuable part of their education.

Here are practical thoughts for everyday poise:

- Posture is one of the first things people notice about you. You can ruin your body's profile by slouching. Keep your back straight and aligned. Your posture should always be regal. With trained muscles, you develop an awareness of the way your body moves. And, since your newfound strength allows you to do things easily, your natural walk appears effortless.

  Perfect posture becomes second nature when you isolate certain muscles and practice simple techniques: Strong abdominal muscles hold your torso and create a solid core or center. Hold your shoulders back slightly, look straight ahead, and keep your back aligned and hands and feet under control.

  When we were growing up, our grandmother Stanley used to tell us to pretend that one end of a silver chain was attached to the breastbone (the sternum) and the other end to a star. When we walked, the silver chain would pull us up and along. Dancers say to imagine the body is a puppet with a string pulling the head to the sky. Either way you feel most comfortable, beautiful posture makes you graceful, youthful, slender, and poised.

- Be aware of your facial expressions and gestures. It is perfectly possible to be both animated and controlled.
- Pick up something from the floor. We were taught to keep our knees together and back straight, and to lower our hips to the floor, torso upright.
- Get out of a car with your knees together. This is particularly important when wearing short skirts. To get into a car, sit first, then lift your legs onto the car floor, feet front, keeping your knees together. To get out of the car, reverse the movement, leading with your feet, keeping knees together.
- Help a friend put on his or her jacket. Reciprocate so that you are comfortable with this movement.

- Learn to sit perfectly still. Control nervous tics and repetitive movements. And, if you're wearing a short skirt, learn to sit so that your integrity is not compromised. In ballroom dancing school, girls were taught to cross legs at the ankles, not at the knees. Try a modern adaptation of this and maintain beautiful posture: Slide your buttocks to the back of the chair, place the small of your back against the chair, keep the calves together, and cross the ankles. Place the calves at an angle and tuck your ankles under your chair (or at the base). Graceful, tasteful, feminine, and uncompromising!
- Learn to stand and walk gracefully in front of a group. Study yourself in a mirror.

DEAR FIRM

"I'm striving for my personal best. I can't compete with Cindy Crawford. But I can be the best I can be!"

FRANCES SCOTT, THIRTY-SOMETHING,
registered nurse, Louisville, Kentucky

HEAR AND SEE YOURSELF AS OTHERS DO

Speech and presentation are important aspects of The FIRM lifestyle. We tell women that they need to know how to present themselves to a camera. Regardless of where they end up in this life, what they've learned will play a central role—at business meetings, presentations, even at PTA meetings or family gatherings.

We encourage our instructors to use good diction and to make eye contact, feel comfortable, and be convincing. It is wonderful to acquire confidence.

Make sure your voice level matches the situation. Some people are oblivious to using their "outdoor" voice inside. People are usually comfortable in asking you to speak up, but rarely will they tell you to stop shouting. They'll just find you obnoxious.

Listen to yourself speaking on tape. What don't you like about the way you sound? If you can't fix the problem or make the change on your own, invest in a good diction and grammar coach as many actors, actresses, and business people do.

As you feel more comfortable in your body, it will be easier to project confidence. And if you practice exuding confidence, you will soon be doing it naturally.

AWAKEN YOUR SENSE OF ADVENTURE

Setting goals means striking out on an adventure. There are, however, two different kinds of adventure. There's the unplanned adventure where you really don't think about where you're going, and you do something wild and crazy. We recommend the other kind of adventure, which is carefully planned and involves taking risks. In this adventure, you push the envelope. You push yourself. The reward is personal growth.

As you reach a new level of physical confidence, you'll want to establish new goals and develop new skills, like going back to school to finish that degree or daring to go whitewater rafting with friends.

Make a commitment to increase your activities and to do new things. As you broaden your scope, you'll further increase your confidence. Just get out and do it—you'll meet people and make new friends. And dare to be unconventional.

DEAR FIRM

"I really believe The FIRM workouts have reversed the aging process in me. I'll be forty in October, and people tell me I look like I'm in my late twenties, early thirties."

AUDREY GREGORY, 39,
office manager/administrative assistant, Palmdale, California

DISCOVER GROUP DANCING

We've always thought of group workouts as a modern form of couples or ballroom dancing. You see, throughout history, dancing has been one of the few activities in which women could express themselves as equals to men.

CHRISTA SUGGS

AGE: 25
PROFESSION: PSYCHOLOGY GRADUATE DEGREE,
MASTERS IN PUBLIC HEALTH

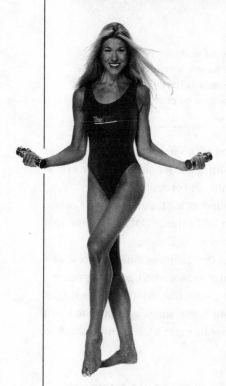

Lovely, blonde Christa has always been very close to her successful, influential mother and as a result was often guided toward specific life and career goals. Christa came to The FIRM without her mother's guidance, but with her own ambition solidly in place.

Christa had been a ballet/jazz dancer and was unhealthily thin. In fact, when she wanted to become an instructor, staff trainer Tracie Long informed her that she was too thin. As Christa tells it, "That's when I realized you look great being healthy. Through The FIRM I gained muscle and became an instructor. That's how I evolved. I feel I gained my womanhood. I learned to be moderate with my exercising and not be excessive."

Then something truly amazing happened: Christa's mother came to The FIRM of her own volition, even taking Christa's class. It was the hardest class Christa had ever taught. And her mom's reaction was an even bigger surprise. Christa reflects, "I felt like, okay, she's going to tell me what I need to do, what I need to say, but she didn't say anything. She's very proud of me. It was weird, though, because I felt like I was over her in a way. That was the first time in my life I felt that way."

Christa's brother, a twenty-six-year-old athlete, also stopped by to check Christa out and had an equally positive reaction. Christa is the first to admit that "The FIRM has done a lot for my family!"

(continued)

But The FIRM has also done a lot for Christa, who recently purchased her own condo. Separating from her family without alienating them, and working to decide on her own career goals are true signs of inner strength, determination, and maturity.

CHRISTA'S TIPS FOR BEGINNERS:
○ If you feel beautiful about yourself, the world will see it.
○ Set your own goals—don't let others (even loved ones) set them for you.
○ We're all looking for ways to maintain self-control; exercise is one of the best, as long as it doesn't become an obsession.

So group exercise classes are an extension of this freedom. Both exercise and dance provide the opportunity for socializing and for moving in time to music. All kinds of dance teach poise, posture, and presentation.

If you want to further improve your dancing technique, take a course in ballroom, shag, or line dancing, or join a dance club. You'll find that these lessons will build confidence in any social situation.

As for which style to try, remember that ballroom dancing is based on the best traditions of European and Latin society, where good manners are prized. While dance trends come and go, you'll find that classic dance styles are always adaptable and in perfect taste. If you are lucky enough to find a man or woman who can dance, you may be in for a terrific romance. And it's a great workout, too!

BECOME AN ACCOMPLISHED HOSTESS

Being a good hostess is a skill as well as an art. Learn the basics by hostessing a small gathering; this will prepare you to handle larger social groups. A good etiquette or entertaining book will provide useful guidelines. Rules are liberating because, once you know them, you are free to make your own. Some tried-and-true entertaining tips:

- Find and brew the best quality coffees and teas.
- Serve top-quality wines and spirits. (They're good social facilitators *in moderation.*)

- Set a lovely table with fresh flowers and good china and linen. Shop secondhand at antique stores for interesting linens, tea services, and flatware. You can even find sterling silver in newspaper classifieds.

BE AN INTERESTING GUEST

It is your responsibility as a guest to participate in pleasant and interesting conversation. During social occasions, try to talk to as many people as you can. Make a special effort to introduce yourself and talk to new people. To prepare for a life in politics, the Kennedy children were taught to be prepared to discuss three current events each night at the supper table. Before your next dinner party, try reading two or three magazines or national newspapers for current topics. You might surprise yourself!

Whatever the occasion, groom and dress yourself with extra effort for evening engagements.

Never comment on another's clothing or possessions. Instead, compliment the other person's attractiveness, achievement, or style.

Restrict the need to talk about yourself. Focus on the other person while in conversation and assist the full development of their ideas. Edit your thoughts and avoid the temptation to digress into extraneous comments. The best conversation is an active exchange of listening and responding.

Perhaps give a small gift to the host/hostess, either when you arrive or afterward, as a thank you. Be sure to thank him/her before you leave and follow up with a thank-you note, call, or fax.

WIT ALWAYS WINS!

Humor is a surefire way to captivate, even in the dark. Innuendo and puns are subtle and, therefore, different from buffoonery. Wit is quietly clever; coarse laughter is barbaric. Our mother tells a story about how she didn't marry a man because of his loud laugh. Perhaps her musical background made her overly sensitive to noise (as opposed to sound), but we believe she shared others' unease in the presence of boorishness, and viewed her ex-beau's behavior as thoughtless and crude.

"I started The FIRM because I wanted to change the way my body LOOKED. I continue because of the way my body FEELS as well as the health benefits. I love working out with The FIRM, and that makes it easy to stay motivated. I feel I can conquer the world—I am Fearless!"

LYNN TYLER, THIRTY-SOMETHING,
professional artist and instructor, Manchester, New Hampshire

FIND A MENTOR,
LEARN FROM ROLE MODELS

When the young peasant Rudolf Nureyev began his dance career in Russia, he lived with an older couple; the woman taught him how to dance, and her husband taught him social graces. A mentor is usually someone you know who helps you learn something about life, about yourself, or both. The fun part is that you don't even have to let the person know they're your mentor. Just watch and learn. At The FIRM, we train our instructors in mentoring the people in their classes and in serving as role models, both in the studio and on the videotapes. This can make a crucial difference, especially for beginners, in their attitude toward the program.

Don't ever be afraid to copy the looks and styles of others you admire, since you'll be adding your unique education, point of view, and ethics to the package.

When you yourself become a mentor or role model, realize your responsibility to make the other person feel good about himself or herself. That's really what life is all about: What makes you feel wonderful about yourself is taking care of other people's needs. Try your best to be kind.

As we've said, most gyms are very hostile, competitive places. We at The FIRM want to be different, which is why we stress kindness in training our instructors, hoping it will pass down to the students. FIRM instructors respect the fact that we all come in different packages with different abilities, and that they are there to assist and help people get where they want to go. They may give a ferocious workout, but instructors always make sure to be gentle with students before and after class. Gentleness to others is an indication of self-confidence.

PERFECT YOUR INNER STYLE

Unique inner beauty can be cultivated by all people through intelligent application, individual style, and selfless charm.

Seize thirty minutes each day for reading nonfiction, especially so-called self-help books. Many of them have actually changed people's lives. When you're driving to work, slip a motivational audiotape into the deck instead of music. Use this information to form opinions about contemporary topics that pertain to your life. Be curious, seek out new knowledge. Goals, truths, and moral principles incubate and are nurtured in this fashion.

Express your opinions publicly only after you have thought them out. Don't rely on TV or other people's ideas to feed you adequate facts. For in-depth coverage and varying points of view, read multiple sources such as newspapers, magazines, and books; then make up your own mind on the subject.

Develop your spiritual life—whether this means regularly attending church or synagogue, yoga meditation, studying belief systems other than your own, or using nature as the bridge to an expanded level of universal consciousness. As belief in the self is enhanced by exercise, belief in something greater than that self tends to become a "good habit" many of our students, video clients, and instructors acquire.

Keep a journal including historical data, goal setting, reality checks, and personal essays. Thereby we learn to know our inner and outer selves and to appreciate the nature of change. The Daily Planner template in chapter 7 will show you how to start.

Create a personal library. All such collections of important source materials are highly individualistic. Use Anna and Cynthia's suggested source materials (listed at the end of the book) as a starting point for your own collection, which will change over time and reflect your own evolution.

Never stop learning! Anna spent a year reading the eleventh edition of the *Encyclopedia Britannica*. Then she studied Greek sculpture and Greek history. She's been actively reading and simultaneously watching the verbatim BBC productions of Shakespeare for the past two years.

"Feeling good about how I look gives me confidence in all areas of my life. Doing The FIRM is a great stress reliever. It's a great physical and emotional 'uplift.' I don't know how I got by without it."

VANESSA SKYM, THIRTY-SOMETHING,
computer operator, St. Johns, Michigan

FIRM PRINCIPLES

To sum up: The FIRM provides a foundation for the rest of life. It is not intended to be a substitute for life. Regular compulsories result in good health and an injury- and pain-free existence. Basic fitness creates the strength to do the things that really matter, such as working hard and thinking hard.

Doing new things and going new places takes energy. It takes a lively readiness to rise above the mundane nature of most chores. Walking down the street in the hot sun, participating in active sports, traveling, doing yardwork, carrying groceries or children all require gusto. You've got to have stamina to enjoy long and late romantic interludes.

Our mother told us, "You have to take care of yourself. If you don't, no one else will." By caring for our bodies and our minds, we are more capable of establishing healthy relationships. Life becomes a gratifying, loving, and rewarding experience.

We at The FIRM know that this state of heightened well-being is possible for you, no matter what your weight, age, or shape. Work out regularly, eat sensibly, never stop learning, and you truly can look forward to becoming the best that you can be!

CHAPTER 7

FIRM
resolve

Welcome to The FIRM Daily Planner, a priceless organizational tool that has helped countless instructors, clients, and FIRM Believers get with—and stick with—the program. Both of us have seen how keeping the journal boosts results, so we swear by it.

In this section we're supplying you with sample pages that will guide you to a new and stronger body and mind. Use these sample pages as a model for your own journal so that you will have a monthly, ongoing record of your progress toward your goals. By letting The FIRM Daily Planner become your personal trainer, you can expect to reach your personal best in record time!

For each day, you'll keep track of your life using four forms: (1) The Health and Work Scheduler, (2) The Diet Analyzer, (3) The Workout Inventory, and (4) The Personality Snapshot. We also supply you with three healthy, satisfying sample Daily Diets and a comprehensive listing of Food Counts to making analyzing your diet easier.

At the end of the month, you can review the pages of your journal, look for patterns and food triggers, and chart your progress. Just by writing things down, reviewing and studying what you eat, and keeping track of your workout schedule and emotional state you can learn a lot about yourself—what you're doing wrong as well as right—and really motivate yourself!

The Health and Work Scheduler

Here's where you organize your day, incorporating fitness with the rest of your activities.

- The *Dayplanner* section helps you arrange your day and maximize each hour's potential.
- The *To Do* section can be used to list your personal and work goals in addition to the Health Goals already listed. When you have accomplished a goal, simply check it off.
- *Health Goals* lists fitness objectives you should try to meet every day. Check them off as you accomplish them—but remember, be honest!
- The *Ratio Chart* is the Scheduler's most crucial element; it summarizes information from the Diet Analyzer page. Its pie chart displays the ideal ratio of daily nutritional intake: 55–65 percent carbohydrates, 20–25 percent protein, and 15–20 percent fat. Through daily analysis of your diet, you'll memorize this ratio!
- The *Notes/Contacts* section provides extra space in which to jot down names, telephone numbers, and/or daily reminders.

HEALTH & WORK SCHEDULER   Day_____   Date_____

DAYPLANNER
Include fitness activities.

7:00

8:00

9:00

10:00

11:00

12:00

1:00

2:00

3:00

4:00

5:00

6:00

7:00

NOTES/CONTACTS

TO DO
Personal/Work Goals   ✓

○

○

○

○

○

○

HEALTH GOALS   ✓

Drink 64 oz. of water.............................. ○

Do some form of exercise...................... ○

Right caloric intake................................. ○

Right carb/protein/fat ratio..................... ○

No junk food.. ○

CALCULATE YOUR RATIO
Enter your food percentages from the Diet Analyzer.

Fat (15–20% Ideal)...

Protein (20–25% Ideal)..

Carbohydrate (55–65% Ideal).................

PROTEIN
20-25%

FAT
15-20%

CARBOHYDRATE
55-65%

The Diet Analyzer

Here you'll keep a complete record of everything—and we *mean* everything—you eat. At the end of the day, you can discover (through some simple math) how much of your diet consists of protein and carbohydrates, and then transfer them to the Health and Work Scheduler to compare them with the ideal ratio.

Keeping a food diary is an absolute necessity for improving your diet. But you must commit to telling the absolute truth! Honesty is all. Even when the diary is to be totally private, a staggering number of people just plain lie—or skip entries because "it was just half of a friend's candy bar, so it didn't count"! Give yourself permission to admit mistakes in your diet. (Isolating problems is, after all, the goal.) Focus on the important components of a healthy diet without obsessing about overly exact portions and precise calorie counts. You can benefit from the diary without filling in every blank every day.

Most of us have a general idea of what we should be eating and when we're breaking the rules. But virtually everyone underestimates caloric intake.

Most of us have little idea how much food we put on our plates. "That little carton of Häagen-Dazs is the biggest joke in the grocery store," says comedienne Elaine Boozler. "It says it serves four people!" Most calorie charts list "calories per 4-ounce serving." That's one-half cup. Practice with a measuring cup so you can visualize this quantity, estimate serving sizes, and approximate calories.

Most of us cycle between two states: starving and bingeing. A regular schedule of five small meals a day can stop this destructive pattern. By keeping your body fueled throughout the day, this practice prevents severe between-meal drops in blood sugar and the resulting ravenous hunger that makes portion control impossible.

○ For each meal, record your food, portion size, estimated amount of calories, protein grams, and fat grams. Add these to create subtotals for each of your meals.

○ At the end of the day, combine the subtotals to find your grand total of calories, protein grams, and fat grams. Then follow these simple steps, noted with the corresponding numbers on the sample page:

DIET ANALYZER

Day_____ **Date**_____

Food/Serving Size	Calories	Protein (g)	Fat (g)
1 MEAL			
1 MEAL SUBTOTAL			
2 MINI-MEAL			
2 MINI-MEAL SUBTOTAL			
3 MEAL			
3 MEAL SUBTOTAL			
4 MINI-MEAL			
4 MINI-MEAL SUBTOTAL			
5 MEAL			
5 MEAL SUBTOTAL			

GRAND TOTAL	Total Calories	Total Protein	Total Fat

Subtract protein and fat percentages from 100 to find carbohydrate percentage, then enter your ratio on the **Health & Work Scheduler** page.

x 4 — Protein Cal. **=**

x 10 — Fat Cal. **=**

÷ (Total Cal) (Total Cal)

% Protein **=**   % Fat **=**

Insert these totals at left.

100 - [% Protein] **-** [% Fat] **=** [% Carbohydrates]

1. Multiply your total protein grams by four and your fat grams by ten to find protein calories and fat calories.

2. Divide these figures by your total number of calories to find the protein and fat percentages of your total nutritional intake. (Remember to move the decimal point two places to the right when converting to a percentage!)

3. Subtract protein and fat percentages from one hundred to find your carbohydrate percentage. You may now transfer these percentages to the Health and Work Scheduler page.

The Workout Inventory

This form keeps detailed records of each of your workouts.

If you use FIRM videos as your workout, note them in the space provided and check off the appropriate intensity level.

If you work out with weights (either in a gym or at home), use the Weight Training Log to keep track of sets, reps, and poundage.

If you complement your workouts with some sort of aerobic activity or cross train, note this in the Aerobic Activity column, including the length of time spent doing the activity and how hard you worked.

Intensity of an activity is your level of exertion in performing that activity. For example, a leisurely walk may be considered light intensity, a brisk walk including a few hills may be moderately intense, while a run may be extremely intense.

Base your level of intensity on your ability to carry on a conversation. If you can speak regularly, you are at a low intensity; a few sentences at a time would be considered moderately intense; and if you can only say a few words, your level is extremely intense.

Finally, rate your Endorphin Levels prior to and after your workout. Endorphins are natural hormones that reduce pain and cause feelings of exhilaration. A good workout stimulates endorphin production.

WORKOUT INVENTORY

Day_____ **Date**_____

VIDEOS/AUDIOS

	Duration (Minutes)	Intensity		
		Light	Moderate	Hard
....		○ ○	○ ○	○
....		○ ○	○ ○	○
....		○ ○	○ ○	○

WEIGHT TRAINING

		Set 1	Set 2	Set 3	Set 4
1	**WEIGHT**				
	REPS				
2	**WEIGHT**				
	REPS				
3	**WEIGHT**				
	REPS				
4	**WEIGHT**				
	REPS				
5	**WEIGHT**				
	REPS				
6	**WEIGHT**				
	REPS				
7	**WEIGHT**				
	REPS				
8	**WEIGHT**				
	REPS				
9	**WEIGHT**				
	REPS				
10	**WEIGHT**				
	REPS				
11	**WEIGHT**				
	REPS				

AEROBIC ACTIVITY

	Duration (Minutes)	Intensity		
		Light	Moderate	Hard
....		○ ○	○ ○	○

ENDORPHIN LEVELS

Pre-Workout			Post-Workout		
Low	Medium	High	Low	Medium	High
○ ○	○ ○	○	○ ○	○ ○	○

The Personality Snapshot

The Personality Snapshot forms should be completed each day, preferably at bedtime. Rate yourself in each of the categories listed, adding specific notes as necessary. Here again, honesty is key!

As you begin to familiarize yourself with each scale, try to define your "neutral zone" (around five) as a "standard" day with no extremes. As you move through the challenges of your program, expect fluctuations in each scale. Take note of conspicuous drops and lifts. Generally, there is an identifiable reason for such fluctuations. Discovering it can help you successfully modify future behavior.

Done daily, The Personality Snapshot will give you, in black and white, an overview of your personal patterns: a visual image that sticks in the mind. By the end of the month, you'll remember the impact of each aspect on the others and the general relationship between them—even when you're no longer charting your workouts or caloric intake. In all areas of your life, you'll have the awareness and knowledge to make the healthiest of lifestyle choices.

You'll see how one dimension of fitness affects another: rest and recovery rate, diet and mood, self-esteem and body image. You'll realize the strong correlation between self-image and weight, diet quality, exercise intensity, and rest. Workout results also influence self-image and emotions. Emerging personal patterns will be shocking and profound. These graphs show you things about yourself that years of psychotherapy could not uncover!

The Daily Diets

To get you started toward healthy eating habits, the following pages contain three days of sample meals that you can plug into your Diet Analyzer. Feel free to mix and match meals to suit your taste. And remember: It's often best to plan your meals in advance to ensure you'll meet the 60:25:15 percent carbohydrate/protein/fat ratio!

PERSONALITY SNAPSHOT   Day_____   Date_____

DIET

Notes ....
Hunger levels, binges, quantity & quality control (portion size, fast foods, restaurant meals), medications, allergens, vitamin/mineral supplements.

1	2	3	4	5	6	7	8	9	10
empty calories		low quality		average			nutrient-dense		clean

WORKOUT

Notes ....
Energy level and reserve, amount of exertion, practice, proficiency, plateaus, technique, mastery of skills, degree of difficulty, satisfaction, dread, proper degree of control.

1	2	3	4	5	6	7	8	9	10
sluggish		weak		average			productive		dynamic

RECOVERY

Notes ....
Injury, fatigue, pain, soreness, stiffness, joint mobility, insomnia, sleep deprivation, naps, meditation or deep relaxation, alternative physical activities.

1	2	3	4	5	6	7	8	9	10
injury		weak		average			strong		powerful

EMOTIONS

Notes ....
Mood swings, stress, pressures, negativity, pessimism, optimism, expectations, challenges, hopes, fears, tenacity, failures, pleasures, satisfaction, fulfillment, defeats, victories, contentment.

1	2	3	4	5	6	7	8	9	10
depressed		unhappy		neutral			happy		elated

INTELLECT

Notes ....
Creativity, evolution, change, goals, organization and preparation, strategies, inspirations, original thoughts, relaxation, habits, perseverance, tactics, expectations, problem-solving, wisdom, knowledge.

1	2	3	4	5	6	7	8	9	10
dull		slow		average			original		sharp

SELF IMAGE

Notes ....
Purpose, center, accountability, reconciliation, self-confidence, self-image, positive feedback, assertiveness, boldness, self-control, discipline, visualization, personal style, inner peace.

1	2	3	4	5	6	7	8	9	10
negative		critical		neutral			accepting		personal best

WEIGHT

Today's Weight .... **Starting weight** ....

Weigh every day in the morning before breakfast. Plot your weight losses and gains relative to your starting weight (SW). Weight loss should be limited to 4-6 pounds per month. Muscle (not fat) weight gain should be limited to about 1 pound per month.

-7	-6	-5	-4	-3	-2	-1	SW	+1	+2

TRANSFER YOUR RATINGS TO THE PERSONALITY PROFILE BOOKMARK

DAILY DIET #1

Food/Serving Size	Calories	Protein (g)	Fat (g)
1 MEAL Oatmeal, 8 oz.	145		2.5
Scrambled eggs (4 whites + 1 yolk)	155	22	
Orange, 1	65		
Flaxseed (on Oatmeal), 2 tsp.	35		2.5
1 MEAL SUBTOTAL	400	22	5
2 MINI-MEAL Yogurt, non-fat, 8 oz.	110	11	
Banana, 1	105		
Pumpkin seeds, 1 oz.	130		6
2 MINI-MEAL SUBTOTAL	345	11	6
3 MEAL Green beans, 8 oz.	50		
Brown rice, 8 oz.	200		1
Lean ground beef, 3 oz.	220	21	10
3 MEAL SUBTOTAL	470	21	11
4 MINI-MEAL Protein powder, 2 scoops	130	13	
Strawberries, 10	50		
Yogurt, non-fat 8 oz.	110	11	
Ice			
4 MINI-MEAL SUBTOTAL	290	24	0
5 MEAL Baked apple, 1	80		.5
Chicken 3 oz., garlic 1 oz., olive oil, 1/2tbsp.	207	26	7
Kale, 8 oz.	40		1
New potatoes with seasonings, 9 oz.	155		
Pineapple, 2 oz.	20		
5 MEAL SUBTOTAL	502	26	8.5

GRAND TOTAL	Total Calories	Total Protein	Total Fat
	2007	104	30.5

	x 4	**x 10**
	Protein Cal.	Fat Cal.
	= 416	= 305

Subtract protein and fat percentages from 100 to find carbohydrate percentage, then enter your ratio on the **Health & Work Scheduler** page.

	÷ 2007 (Total Cal)	2007 (Total Cal)
	% Protein	% Fat
	= 21	= 15

100 - | % Protein | - | % Fat | = | % Carbohydrates |
| 21 | | 15 | | 64 |

Insert these totals at left.

DAILY DIET #2

Food/Serving Size	Calories	Protein (g)	Fat (g)
1 MEAL Pancakes, 2 medium	200	4	6
Maple syrup, 2 tbsp.	100		
Low-fat ham, 3 oz.	100	17	2
Grapefruit, 1/2	46		
1 MEAL SUBTOTAL	446	21	8
2 MINI-MEAL Yogurt, non-fat 8 oz.	110	11	
Fresh fruit, 6 oz.	100		
Pumpkin seeds, 1 oz.	130		6
2 MINI-MEAL SUBTOTAL	340	11	6
3 MEAL Tuna, 3 oz.	100	21	1
Brown rice, 6 oz.	150		2
Salad, 8 oz.	80		
Carrots, 4 oz.	44		1
3 MEAL SUBTOTAL	374	21	4
4 MINI-MEAL Pear, 1	95		
Cottage cheese, non-fat, 6 oz.	135	18	
Muffin, 1	175		6
4 MINI-MEAL SUBTOTAL	405	18	6
5 MEAL Pasta, 6 oz.	150		1
Chicken, 3 oz., garlic, 1 oz., olive oil, 1/2 tbsp.	207	26	7
Grated romano cheese, 2 tbsp.	40	4	6
Squash and spinach, 4 oz. each	55		
Tomato and onions w/seasonings, 4 oz.	100		
5 MEAL SUBTOTAL	552	30	14
GRAND TOTAL	**Total Calories** 2117	**Total Protein** 101	**Total Fat** 38

Subtract protein and fat percentages from 100 to find carbohydrate percentage, then enter your ratio on the **Health & Work Scheduler** page.

	x 4	**x 10**
	Protein Cal.	Fat Cal.
	= 404	= 380
	÷ 2117 *(Total Cal)*	2117 *(Total Cal)*
	% Protein	% Fat
	= 19	= 18

Insert these totals at left.

100 - | % Protein 19 | **-** | % Fat 18 | **=** | % Carbohydrates 63 |

DAILY DIET #3

Food/Serving Size	Calories	Protein (g)	Fat (g)
1 MEAL Cantelope, 8 oz.	60		
Tuna, water packed, 3 oz.	100	21	1
Toast, 2 pieces	140		
Fruit-only jam, 2 tsp.	28		
1 MEAL SUBTOTAL	328	21	1
2 MINI-MEAL Yogurt, non-fat, 8 oz.	110	11	
Grapefruit, 1/2	46		
Cherries, 4 oz.	60		
Turkey, 3 oz.	134	25	3
2 MINI-MEAL SUBTOTAL	350	36	3
3 MEAL Baked chicken, 3 oz.	150	20	4
Cooked beets w/vinegar, 4 oz.	46		
Brown rice, 4 oz.	100		1
Broccoli, 4 oz.	24		
Peach, 1	37		
3 MEAL SUBTOTAL	357	20	5
4 MINI-MEAL Tuna, 3 oz.	100	21	1
Rice cakes, 3	120		
Celery and carrots, 4 oz. each	56		
Pumpkin seeds, 1 oz.	127		5.5
4 MINI-MEAL SUBTOTAL	403	21	6.5
5 MEAL Lean ground beef, 3oz.	220	21	10
Fresh pineapple, 4 oz.	40		
Sweet potato, 1 medium	136		
Green beans, 4 oz.	17		
Watermelon, 1" by 10" slice	152		2
5 MEAL SUBTOTAL	565	21	12

GRAND TOTAL	Total Calories	Total Protein	Total Fat
	2003	122	38.5

	x 4	x 10
	Protein Cal.	Fat Cal.
	= 488	= 385

Subtract protein and fat percentages from 100 to find carbohydrate percentage, then enter your ratio on the **Health & Work Scheduler** page.

÷ 2003   2003
(Total Cal)   (Total Cal)

	% Protein	% Fat
	= 24	= 19

100 - | % Protein | - | % Fat | = | % Carbohydrates |
| 24 | | 19 | | 57 |

Insert these totals at left.

Food Counts

It's not hard to analyze your diet if you eat simple, nutritious foods. Cooking and processing, as you know, destroy some, and sometimes all, of the nutritional quality of foods, so build your diet around things as close to the natural, raw state as possible.

The following food counts are included because they are commonly listed as foods frequently eaten by successful athletes. The potential list of good foods is much larger than can easily be encompassed here. So you may want to refer to a more encyclopedic source, such as the recently updated *The Complete Book of Food Counts* by Corinne T. Netzer, published by Dell in 1997.

Note on protein: While some plants and vegetables contain protein, they are *incomplete* proteins and have to be combined with complementary carbohydrates that are sources of the missing amino acids. Proteins from animal sources are complete; they have all nine of the essential amino acids the body needs to repair muscle tissue. *Food Counts* only lists protein values for sources of *complete proteins.*

PROTEIN: DAIRY

Include these foods because most are high in the essential mineral calcium and are good protein sources. All dairy foods are high in fat, unless low-fat or non-fat varieties are selected. Many semi-vegetarian diets substitute egg whites and yogurt for meats. Lactose and egg-intolerant individuals can compensate by substituting more meat for dairy products and taking calcium supplements. Important dairy sources to remember: eggs (or egg whites), yogurt.

Food	Serving	Calories	Protein(g)	Fat(g)
Cheese, grated				
Parmesan or Romano	1 tblsp.	23	2	2
Cheese, Farmer	2 oz.	50	4	4
Cottage Cheese, non-fat	2 oz.	45	6	0
Egg				
white	1	17	4	0
whole	1	75	6	5
Milk				
non-fat	8 oz.	90	9	0
1% fat	8 oz.	100	8	2
Protein Powder	2 scoops	130	13	
Yogurt, plain, non-fat	8 oz.	110	11	0

PROTEIN: MEATS

Meats, together with seafood and dairy, are the foundation of each meal of the day. These foods also contain vitamin B12, a builder of red blood cells, which is particularly important for bodybuilders. All meats are high in fat unless low-fat or non-fat varieties are selected. All 3 ounce portions contain approximately the same number of calories and a complete serving of protein. Important meat sources to remember: chicken and ground round, 3 oz. portions.

Food	Serving	Calories	Protein(g)	Fat(g)
Beef, ground				
broiled, extra-lean	3 oz.	218	22	10
Chicken				
dark meat, no skin	3 oz.	174	23	8
light meat, no skin	3 oz.	147	26	4
light meat, with skin	3 oz.	190	20	11
Ham				
lean (2% fat)	4 oz.	130	23	3
Pork, fat-trimmed	3 oz.	218	24	13

PROTEIN: MEATS *(continued)*

Food	Serving	Calories	Protein(g)	Fat(g)
Sirloin, Top				
broiled, fat-trimmed	3 oz.	172	26	7
Turkey				
light meat, no skin	3 oz.	134	25	3

PROTEIN: SEAFOOD

Seafoods are an interesting and diverse protein source and, unlike land animals, are basically low in fat unless cooking oils are added. All 3 ounce portions contain approximately the same number of calories and a complete serving of protein. Important seafood source to remember: water-packed canned tuna.

Food	Serving	Calories	Protein(g)	Fat(g)
Catfish	4 oz.	132	21	5
Caviar, granular	1 tblsp.	40	4	3
Clams				
raw, large	9	133	23	2
raw, small	20	133	23	2
steamed	4 oz.	168	29	2
Cod, broiled, baked	4 oz.	119	26	1
Crab				
Alaskan King	4 oz.	96	21	1
Blue	4 oz.	100	20	1
Dungeness	4 oz.	96	20	1
Queen, raw	4 oz.	104	21	1
Crab, "imitation"	4 oz.	116	14	2
Grouper, baked or broiled	4 oz.	134	28	2
Halibut, baked or broiled	4 oz.	159	30	3
Lobster, boiled or steamed	4 oz.	111	23	1
Salmon, Pink				
baked, broiled	4 oz.	245	31	12
canned in water	4 oz.	140	20	6
Shrimp, boiled	4oz.	112	24	1
Sole, baked or broiled	4 oz.	133	27	2
Tuna				
fresh	4 oz.	164	26	6
canned in water	3 oz.	100	21	1

CARBOHYDRATES: STARCHY

Ideally, about half of your daily carbohydrate allotment (about 600 calories) should come from this category. They are of optimal nutritional value when they are unrefined and unprocessed, as nature made them. Important starchy carbs to remember: baked potatoes, brown rice, and oatmeal.

Food	Serving	Calories	Fat(g)
Bagel	2 oz.	150	1
Baked Potato	1 med.	220	< 1
Beans			
black	4 oz.	113	1
black-eyed peas	4 oz.	100	1
lentils	4 oz.	115	0
pinto	4 oz.	117	< 1
Bread			
wheat, pita	1 whole	150	2
wheat, slice	1 slice	70	1
Biscuit	1	100	1
Bulgur	8 oz.	152	< 1
Cereal			
bran	1 oz.	90	< 1
Couscous	1 oz.	107	< 1
Granola	1 oz.	130	4
Grits, cooked	1 cup	146	1
Melba Toast	6 pieces	100	
Millet, cooked	4 oz.	135	1
Muffin, home-made	6 oz.	175	6
New potato, boiled	4 oz.	68	
Oatmeal	8 oz.	145	2
Pasta, dry, cooked	8 oz.	197	1
Rice Cakes	1	40	< 1
Rice			
brown	4 oz.	100	1
white	4 oz.	103	< 1
Sweet Potato	1 med.	136	< 1

CARBOHYDRATES: FIBROUS

Ideally, about 3 to 5 servings (about 200 calories) of your daily carbohydrate intake should come from this category. Note the large quantity of these vitamin and mineral-rich foods you must eat to consume 200 calories. They are of optimal nutritional value when they are unrefined, unprocessed, and raw. Important fibrous carbs to remember: carrots, beets, kale, broccoli, and cabbage.

Food	Serving	Calories	Fat(g)
Asparagus, spears	3.8 oz.	13	0
Bean Sprouts	2 oz.	6	0
Beets, fresh	4 oz.	40	< 1
Bok Choy, raw	4 oz.	5	< 1
Broccoli, spears	4oz.	24	< 1
Brussel Sprouts, boiled	4 oz.	30	< 1
Cabbage			
white, raw, shredded	4 oz.	8	< 1
red, raw, shredded	4 oz.	10	< 1
Carrots, raw	4 oz.	44	< 1
Cauliflower	4 oz.	15	< 1
Celery, stalks	1.6 oz.	6	0
Corn, kernels	4 oz.	89	1
Cucumber	1 medium	39	< 1
Green Beans	4 oz.	17	0
Greens			
kale	4 oz.	21	< 1
mustard	4 oz.	11	< 1
romaine lettuce	4 oz.	4	< 1
spinach	4 oz.	21	< 1
swiss chard	4 oz.	18	1
Mushrooms, raw	4 oz.	9	< 1
Onions, raw	4 oz.	44	< 1
Okra, boiled	4 oz	25	< 1
Peppers, green or red	4 oz.	30	< 1
Sprouts			
alfalfa, raw	4 oz.	5	< 1
Squash			
butternut, baked	4 oz.	41	< 1
summer, yellow	4 oz.	18	< 1
zucchini, green	4 oz.	14	< 1
Tomatoes	1	26	0

CARBOHYDRATES: FRUITS

Ideally, about 3-5 servings (about 300 calories) of your daily carbohydrate intake come from this category. They contain slightly more calories per serving than fibrous carbohydrates. Because these foods contain sugar, they provide quick energy and are an excellent substitute for starchy carbs. They are of optimal nutritional value when they are eaten raw. Estimate one serving to be approximately 75 calories, and prefer all available sources in season. Important fruits to remember: citrus fruits, melons, apples.

Food	Serving	Calories	Fat(g)
Apple			
raw, w/ peel	1	81	1
raw, peeled	1	72	< 1
dried	2 oz.	145	0
Applesauce, unsweetened	4 oz.	53	< 1
Apricots			
fresh	4 oz.	37	< 1
dried	4 oz.	280	0
Banana, whole	1	105	1
Blackberries, fresh	4 oz.	37	< 1
Blueberries, fresh	4 oz.	41	< 1
Cantelope			
cubed	4 oz.	29	< 1
½ of 5" diameter		94	1
Cherries, fresh	4 oz.	56	< 1
Cranberries			
fresh, whole	4 oz.	23	< 1
canned, sauce	4 oz.	289	< 1
Currants, dried	4 oz.	204	< 1
Figs			
fresh	1	37	< 1
dried	10	477	2
Fruit-only jam	1 tsp.	14	0
Grapes	10	15	< 1
Grapefruit	1/2	46	< 1
Honeydew Melons			
cubed	4 oz.	30	< 1
7" by 2" slice		46	< 1
Kiwifruit	1	46	< 1
Mango	1	54	< 1

CARBOHYDRATES: FRUITS *(continued)*

Food	Serving	Calories	Fat(g)
Nectarine	1	67	1
Orange			
navel, 2½" diameter	1	65	< 1
valencia, 2½" diameter	1	59	< 1
Papaya	4 oz.	27	< 1
Peach			
fresh	1	37	< 1
dried	2 oz.	140	0
Pear, Bartlett	1	98	1
Pineapple, fresh	4 oz.	39	< 1
Plum	1	46	1
Prunes, dried	2 oz.	120	0
Raisins	4 oz.	219	< 1
Raspberries, fresh	4 oz.	31	< 1
Rhubarb, fresh	4 oz.	13	< 1
Strawberries			
fresh	4 oz.	23	< 1
frozen (no sugar)	5 oz.	50	1
Tangerine, fresh	1	37	< 1
Watermelon	1" by 10" slice	152	2

FATS: LUXURY AND ESSENTIAL

These foods are the most dense and concentrated forms of energy: each gram contains more than twice the calories of proteins and carbohydrates. The only fats which are necessary for healthy skin and tissues are the unsaturated fatty acids. Important essential fats to remember: flaxseed and pumpkin seeds.

Food	Serving	Calories	Fat(g)
Avocado	4 oz.	204	20
Canola Oil	1 tblsp.	120	14
Butter	1 tblsp.	34	4
Flaxseed, freshly ground	1 tblsp.	70	5
Nuts/Seeds			
almonds, raw	1 oz.	170	15
pumpkin seeds, raw	1 oz.	127	6
sesame seeds, raw	1 tsp.	16	2
sunflower seeds, raw	1 oz.	160	13
Olive Oil	1 tblsp.	120	14

MISCELLANEOUS

Food	Serving	Calories	Fat(g)
Coffee	6 oz.	4	0
Garlic	1 oz.	42	< 1
Ginger, fresh	1 oz.	20	< 1
Herbs, fresh	1 tsp.	9	1
Horseradish	4 oz.	6	< 1
Maple Syrup	1 tblsp.	50	0
Mustard, Dijon	1 tsp.	8	1
Pepper, ground	1 tsp.	5	0
Sea Salt	1 tblsp.	0	0
Soy Sauce	1 tsp.	< 1	0
Vinegar			
balsamic	1 tblsp.	1	0
cider	1 tblsp.	2	0
red wine	1 tblsp.	6	0
white wine	1 tblsp.	4	0

Bon Voyage

Armed with *FIRM for Life* and your Daily Planner, you are about to embark on a voyage of discovery toward a new you—shapelier, healthier, happier, and full of vigor. We at The FIRM know you can realize your dreams, because we've seen and read the letters of so many before you who have attained their goals. Have a wonderful journey!

APPENDIX

ANNA'S SUGGESTED READINGS

A Brief History of Time: From the Big Bang to Black Holes by Stephen W. Hawking
Written by a trailblazing physicist, this book organizes the universe into a meaningful time line.

Caterin' to Charleston by Gloria Mann Maynard and *Charleston Receipts,* collected by The Junior League of Charleston
These books are well-thumbed. I mix and match all of the hot breads. A Southern-based vocabulary of basics upon which you can build Italian and Japanese cuisines.

The Complete Works of William Shakespeare
The beauty and originality of Shakespeare make this the most important book in the English language. He sets the standards and limits of English literature through unparalled use of the language. Shakespeare fuses cognitive acuity, linguistic energy, and power of invention into a profusion of genius. The resulting works are rich and thought-provoking. Delightfully original characters express an enormous capacity for joy and spontaneous delight in the moment.

A Dictionary of Music & Musicians (1450–1889) edited by Sir George Grove
A Victorian compendium of musical geniuses with beautifully written, intimate biographies.

The Encyclopaedia Britannica, a Dictionary of Arts, Sciences, Literature and General Information, Eleventh edition
This revered item is the number one choice for researchers in the European liberal arts. The essays are signed and were written at the turn of the century by the best of the Edwardian scholars of England. Available through used book dealers.

Great Books of the Western World by Encyclopaedia Britannica, Inc.
A compilation of fifty authors, and their works, representing 2,500 years of Western thought, compiled for the first time with a *Synopticon* of 102 ideas that cross reference and index the entire body of knowledge.

The Great Ideas: A Lexicon of Western Thought by Mortimer Adler
Published separately, these are the all-important 102 essays that were originally introduced as the *Synopticon,* the cornerstone of an extensive cross-referencing and indexing system for the Britannica's *Great Books of the Western World.*

The Holy Bible, King James Version
   The definitive text for Western spirituality.

The Home Owners' Complete Garden Handbook by John Hayes Melady
   A Southern text for my native flora, annotated by my mother during our formative years on a small farm in the rural Carolina countryside.

The Inner Game of Tennis by W. Timothy Gallwey
   A wonderful tool for growth and knowledge of the natural self through gamesmanship.

Mandy Tandy's Bodybuilding Nutrition by Mandy Tandy
   Nutrition-packed, high-energy recipes that emphasize natural foods and healthy nutrients.

The Mysterious William Shakespeare
   A passionate and eloquent presentation of Edward de Vere, seventeenth Earl of Oxford, as the true author of the plays and sonnets. The theory is established by demonstrating the astonishing literary and biographical connections between the published works and the life of de Vere. This is a necessary companion to a meaningful study of the works of Shakespeare. Knowledge of the man who wrote the words enhances the literature profoundly.

The Nude, A Study in Ideal Form by Kenneth Clark
   This book reviews the human form using predominantly classical sculpture, which combines beauty and emotions. Superior images of harmony, energy, ecstasy, humility, and pathos illustrate, through nudity, the superiority of the Greeks.

Nutrition and Physical Degeneration: A Comparison of Primitive and Modern Diets and Their Effects by Weston A. Price
   A primer for breeding. Most women devote a lifetime of resources and about ten biological years to this cycle. This task is made easier through the knowledge supplied by this book of the visible effects of inferior and superior diets.

The Seven Habits of Highly Effective People by Stephen R. Covey
   An amazingly powerful self-help book. I preferred the unedited audio-tape version that gives the motivation to tackle the world while you drive into it.

Success Is a Choice: Ten Steps to Overachieving in Business and Life by Rick Pitino
   Bringing the athletic touch to self-improvement, this famous basketball coach (formerly of the Kentucky Wildcats, now of the Boston Celtics) teaches us to reach success through choice, with a strategy of overachieving. Setting high goals, he preaches a no-quit philosophy for developing habits and discipline to make your dreams a reality. This is a ten-step plan of ferocious persistence for winners.

Vogue's Book of Etiquette by Millicent Fenwick
   Written by the associate editor of *Vogue,* this is a period piece that discusses the timeless value of civility. The basic rules always apply. It was a gift from my mother.

The Wheel of Life by Elizabeth Kubler-Ross, M.D.

This book traces the intellectual and spiritual development of a woman who has transformed the way we look at death and dying. Remarkable personal sacrifice and charity has allowed Kubler-Ross to give comfort to those who seek to cope with their own deaths and the deaths of loved ones. In a culture that hides dying, this woman opens up the topic so that we can examine it without fear. She shows, using her life as an example, that free will is our greatest gift and that our most important goal is spiritual evolution. Her life's purpose has been to help others live fully and to express love.

The Zone by Barry Sears, Ph.D.

In this excellent presentation of dietary practices, Sears analyzes food in a way that perfectly complements the lifestyle of athletes. His emphasis on natural unrefined carbohydrates and clean, low-fat protein is the solution for improving health and losing weight.

CYNTHIA'S SUGGESTED READINGS

Reference Books on Nutrition and Diet

Alternative Medicine: The Definitive Guide compiled by The Burton Goldberg Group

An encyclopedic work with an impressive list of contributors and consultants. One thousand pages make this reference book an excellent study tool.

Diet & Nutrition by Rudolph Ballentine, M.D.

Includes sections on ecology, biochemistry, physiology, and pharmacology of nutrition, food, and consciousness. Examines eating patterns of ancient peoples vs. modern society, ayurvedic nutrition, megavitamins, and food allergies.

Earl Mindell's Vitamin Bible by Earl Mindell

This pocket book includes comprehensive listings of vitamins, minerals, and herbs; a Q&A section; and information about finding a nutritionally oriented doctor.

Eat, Drink and Be Healthy by Janet Chiabetta

An easy-to-read book outlining the relationship between diet and disease. Easy-to-understand graphs of dietary fat composition. Recipes and menu planning.

Eight Weeks to Optimum Health by Andrew Weil, M.D.

A comforting and holistic book by bestselling author Weil.

Enzyme Nutrition by Edward Howell

Enzyme theorist Dr. Edward Howell discusses his alternative health approach based on the life force of enzymes.

Fats That Heal, Fats That Kill by Udo Erasmus

A pioneer in new technology for processing healthful oils, Dr. Erasmus has written the definitive work on oils and fats. His research sheds crucial light on the subject of edible oils and their functions, and on modern processing and our nutrition.

Healthy Healing by Linda Rector-Page, N.D., Ph.D.

Another good reference book that recommends for various conditions specific combinations of food, vitamins, herbs, and bodywork.

Nourishing Traditions by Sally Fallon

A comprehensive and sometimes startling cookbook that challenges politically correct nutrition and the diet dictocrats.

Prescription for Nutritional Healing by James F. Balch, M.D. and Phyllis A. Balch, C.N.C.

This encyclopedic work is divided into two primary sections: (1) Understanding the Elements of Health, and (2) The Disorders. Includes comprehensive definitions and dietary/nutritional/herbal recommendations.

Sugar Blues by William Duffy

A modern classic about the history of sugar cultivation and commerce, and the appalling effects on humanity.

Lifestyle/Philosophy

The Book of Good Manners

From the publisher who created a new series for museum bookstores, a clever and insightful illustrated look at the nature of manners and how we all are subject to their influence.

Real Magic by Wayne Dyer

Inspiring book on the power of thought and how to direct our thoughts and actions for spiritual development.

The Road Less Traveled by M. Scott Peck, M.D.

A fresh and original work, Dr. Peck's chapters on love and spirituality have received national praise. He draws no distinction between the process of achieving spiritual growth and achieving mental growth.

Simple Abundance by Sarah Ban Breathnach

Three hundred sixty-six daily essays for spiritual reflections on life, establishing priorities, and confirming our myriad options.

THE FIRM GLOSSARY

The following are fitness buzzwords, concepts that are essential to understanding both diet and exercise. See how many of them you already know.

Abduction   Movement of a body part away from the vertical axis of the body.

Adduction   Movement of a body part toward the vertical axis of the body.

Aerobic training   Exercise that stimulates the cardiovascular system (heart, lungs, blood vessels) through vigorous, sustained activity to provide oxygen to the working muscles.

Anaerobic training   Intense, short-term athletic activity that utilizes stored oxygen in the working muscles. The primary method for increasing muscle strength. Examples include weight training and sprinting.

Bilateral training   Exercises done concurrently that train opposites sides of the body. For example, curling with the right arm while dipping with the left leg.

Calorie   Informally, it's the amount of energy available to (or utilized by) the body. Technically, it is the amount of heat required to raise the temperature of one kilogram of water one degree celsius; also called kilocalorie.

Cheating   A method of pushing a muscle past the point at which it would normally fail. For example, when curling the biceps and you can't quite lift the final reps, you "cheat" by helping ever so slightly with your other hand.

Circuit training   Alternating anaerobic and aerobic total body training using light weights and high repetitions to develop muscle tone, endurance, and cardiovascular fitness.

Compound movement   An exercise that works several muscle groups simultaneously, e.g., lunges work glutes, quads, and gastrocnemius.

Concentric action   Contraction or shortening of a muscle while it is working against resistance.

Eccentric action   Extension or lengthening of a muscle while it is working against resistance.

Endurance   The ability of a muscle to perform a movement repeatedly without fatigue.

Enzyme   Molecules produced by the body that affect the rate of the reactions of the metabolism.

Extension   Increasing the angle of a joint; straightening a joint.

Failure   Complete muscle fatigue that renders further repetitions impossible.

Fitness　The ability to carry out daily tasks with vigor and alertness without undue fatigue and with ample energy to enjoy leisure time and to meet unforeseen emergencies.

Flexion　Decreasing the angle of a joint; bending a joint.

Glycogen　Form of sugar stored in the muscles and the liver. An important first line source of energy during exercise.

High-impact　Movement in which for a split-second neither foot is on the floor.

Hyperextension　Bending backwards beyond the medial line of the joint; creating extreme or excessive extension of the joint.

Interval training　Aerobic training that alternates between periods of intensity (80–85 percent of maximum aerobic capacity) and brief rest (at or just below aerobic threshold).

Isolation movement　An exercise that works only one muscle group; e.g., triceps kickbacks work only the triceps.

Isometric　Resistance training performed without movement.

Isotonic　Resistance training performed with movement through its range of motion.

Lateral movement　Side-to-side exercise that works only one side of the body at a time.

Low-impact　Movement in which one foot remains on the floor.

Medial　Movement toward the midline of the body.

Metabolism　The total of all the processes occurring within the body—including those that build (anabolic) and those that break down (catabolic) tissues.

Minerals　Organic substances needed in the diet to regulate bodily functions. Examples include calcium, sodium, potassium, iron, and selenium.

Muscle confusion　Variations in training schedule in an attempt to "shock" the body out of familiar patterns and into new adaptation, frequently for better results.

Nonimpact　Movement in which both feet remain on the floor.

Nutrient　Metabolic essentials that must be obtained in the diet, including carbohydrates, proteins, fats, water, vitamins, and minerals.

Pre-exhaust　A method of gaining muscle by following an isolation exercise with a general exercise to increase the number of muscle fibers affected.

Prone　Lying on the stomach, face down.

Pyramid　To change the amount of resistance or weight.

Range of motion (ROM)   The degrees of flexion and extension of which a joint is capable.

Repetition   One complete movement of an exercise from start to finish.

Set   A group of repetitions performed continuously, usually followed by a rest interval and then another "set."

Strength   A measure of the ability of a muscle to move an object that resists being moved.

Supine   Lying on the back, face up.

Vertical movement   Up-and-down exercise that works both sides of the body at the same time.

Vitamins   Organic compounds that cannot be manufactured by the body and act as regulators to metabolism. A deficiency of these substances can result in disease.

FIRM DIRECT PRODUCT LIST

•VIDEOS: Follow-Along Workouts

TOTAL BODY
Body Sculpting Basics
Low Impact Aerobics
Aerobic Interval Training
Time Crunch Workout
Abs, Hips & Thighs Sculpting
Complete Aerobic Weight Training

FIRM PARTS
Five Day Abs
Lower Body Sculpting
Standing Legs
Upper Body
Tough Aerobic Mix
Not-So-Tough Aerobics
Five Day Stretch

CROSS TRAINERS
The Tortoise
The Hare
FIRM Cardio
FIRM Strength
Prime Power Fat Burning
Prime Power Lower Body

FIRM BASICS
Sculpting with Weights
Fat Burning
Abs, Buns & Thighs

•VIDEOS: Informational
20 Questions About Fitness
Form Points

•AUDIOS: Follow-Along Workouts
Abs & Pelvic Diaphragm Workout
Easy PowerWalk with Weights
Hard PowerWalk with Weights

•CD-ROM: Informational
The FIRM Personal Fitness

To Place an Order

For a FREE catalog of all FIRM products, call 1-800-THE-FIRM (1-800-843-3476). Mention this book and receive a FREE video with your first order, *20 Questions About Fitness*, a 50-minute video "encyclopedia of fitness," which exposes dozens of myths that *even you* believe. Scientific answers to *all* major body-shaping and fat-loss questions. With 47 animated illustrations, charts, and film clips. You also receive a FREE Workout Guide: *8 Ways to Customize Your Exercise Program*.

FIRM Direct, L.L.C.
Dept. BK
P.O. Box 5716
Columbia, SC 29250-5716

Visit us on the Internet at http://www.firmdirect.com

Send your success stories to:
FIRM Direct, L.L.C.
Department "Success"
P.O. Box 5716
Columbia, SC 29250-5716

The **FIRM**®

EXERCISE VIDEOS FOR ALL LEVELS

Firm Basics
(3 titles)

Classic Workout Series
(6 Total Body titles)   (6 Firm Parts titles)

Cross Trainers
(4 titles)

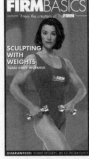

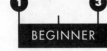

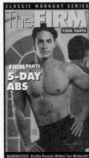

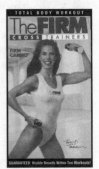

1 — **3** .... **8** — **10**

BEGINNER   INTERMEDIATE   ADVANCED

MORE CHOICES
FROM THE NAME YOU TRUST

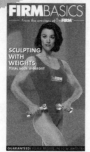
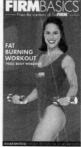
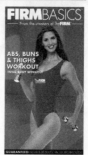

Log of the Mayflower

The Mayflower Compact

In the name of God Amen. We whose names are under-writen, the loyall subjects of our dread soveraigne Lord King James, by the grace of God, of Great Britaine, France, & Ireland, king, defender of the faith, etc. Haveing undertaken, for the glorie of God, and advancemente of the Christian faith and honour of our king & countrie, a voyage to plant the first colonie in the Northerne parts of Virginia, doe by these presents solemnly & mutualy in the presence of God, and one of another, covenant & combine ourselves togeather into a civill body politick, for our better ordering & preservation & furtherance of the ends aforesaid; and by vertue hereof to enacte, constitute, and frame such just & equall lawes, ordinances, acts, constitutions, & offices, from time to time, as shall be thought most meete and convenient for the generall good of the Colonie: unto which we promise all due submission and obedience. In witnes whereof we have hereunder subscribed our names at Cap-Codd the .11. of November, in the year of the raigne of our soveraigne Lord King James of England, France, & Ireland, the eighteenth, and of Scotland the fiftie fourth. Ano:dom. 1620.

John Carver	Samuel Fuller	Edward Tilley
William Bradford	Christopher Martin	John Tilley
Edward Winslow	William Mullins	Francis Cooke
William Brewster	William White	Thomas Rogers
Isaac Allerton	Richard Warren	Thomas Tinker
Myles Standish	John Howland	John Rigdale
John Alden	Stephen Hopkins	Edward Fuller
John Turner	Degory Priest	Richard Clark
Francis Eaton	Thomas Williams	Richard Gardiner
James Chilton	Gilbert Winslow	John Allerton
John Crackston	Edmund Margeson	Thomas English
John Billington	Peter Brown	Edward Dotey
Moses Fletcher	Richard Britteridge	Edward Leister
John Goodman	George Soule	

Log of the Mayflower

by

PHILIP J. SIMON
Author of *Sight Unseen*

Priam Press
CHICAGO, ILLINOIS

Library of Congress Catalog Card Number: 56–9513

———————————

Printed in the United States of America
BY RAND MCNALLY & COMPANY, CHICAGO, ILL.

PILGRIM JOHN HOWLAND

"Hee was a godly man and an ancient professor in the wayes of Christ. Hee was one of the first comers into this land and was the last man that was left of those that came over in the Shipp, called the Mayflower, that lived in Plymouth."

Plymouth Records.

Tuesday, September 5, 1620

God willing and if a fair wind blows on the morrow, the *Mayflower* hoists sail to the breeze and we depart from Plymouth on our voyage to the northern parts of Virginia in America.

Thus with due reverence and solemnity as befits the occasion do I commence this relation of our venture. And truly, considered in the light of all circumstances, it is well calculated to inspire awe in the breast of each of us, from the hoariest Elder to the youngest infant in arms. Here we are, a mere handful, prepared to sail in one small craft over a vast sea to found a settlement in a strange and unknown land. The hazards threatening to assail us are manifold, but for the moment I forbear to say more. Let it suffice to say they loom before us, grim and impassible.

How will it fare with us on the voyage and what will the outcome be? I wish I were gifted with vision to pierce the future and make a proper answer, but that power is denied me. And indeed there is none who can foresee and no one dares attempt to foretell what will come of it. We know we are in the hands of the Almighty and humbly beseech His blessing for the success of our venture. Should it find favor in His eyes, then He will bring us safely to haven despite all obstacles. I pray it be so, and the Lord grant I may live to pen its joyous ending. That which transpired beforehand has trialed us sorely and brought but empty cheer. We had planned to make an earlier departure from England in the hope of arriving at America in the summer or early fall of the year. Had all gone as we planned it, I think we would have been half the sea over by now and well on the way to our journey's end, but we were crossed by adversities which delayed us a full thirty days and more. And now with summer on the wane and the fall season approaching fast we still find ourselves moored to English soil.

The voyage we contemplate is reckoned roundly as one of six weeks' duration. Thus if we should sail on the morrow and cross the sea in safety, we will reach our haven in late October with winter close at hand. This is an appalling prospect, especially when one considers that the wintry seasons there are not to be compared to our English winters. As reports have it, they are notoriously harsh and bitter with biting winds and deadly frosts. How then are we to withstand the rigor and hardship of inclement weather in a strange land where we will be without houses or other means of habitation? I do not know, nor will I at present seek a remedy. When the time comes the Lord will find a way for us if it be His will.

We do not lack faith in Providence, yet it cannot be denied the entire Company is likely to suffer by reason of our departure having been delayed. Indeed it will be

Apart from the dangers attending our belated sailing, the venture bodes ill; if Providence does not lend a helping hand I fear it is foredoomed to disaster. At the outset we are poorly provisioned to dare a voyage of so great an import. Divers merchants in England had pledged to advance us sufficient monies for our needs, but we had a falling out with them concerning the conditions and they refused to keep their bond. This put us in such desperate straits that at Southampton we had to sell almost £100 of our provisions before we could clear the port. We disposed of some five score firkins of butter, and we have no salad oil, shoe leather and other necessaries.

The absence of these needed items might be passed over as not being requisite to the success of our venture, but in addition there is a fatal deficiency in our store of military arms. We are faced with a dearth of armor, cutlasses, swords, snaphances and muskets, and our firearms are matchlocks of an ancient make which are no better than useless in damp weather. With the meager equipment at our command we can scarcely hope to put more than a dozen fully armed men in the field to cope with the multitudes of savages and beasts in the wilds of America.

Secondly, and of more grave concern, unity and concord are woefully lacking in our Company, and if present they would have been welcome friends and allies. Even now dissension is rampant and discord holds sway. The people are at swords' ends with every man ready to fly at his fellow's throat, doubts and misgivings are rife, and the fires of suspicion smolder softly and await the coming of the wind of adversity to burst into flame and consume all. But of this I shall make a fuller relation at some other date.

Thus briefly have I set forth our present condition. Truly it appears desperate, yet not hopeless. Our Leyden people were reared in the uses of adversity, having borne the yoke for many years as exiles in Holland. They are courageous and mightily inspired to brave the perils of the treacherous sea and the hazards of a barbarous land so they may worship God as their conscience governs. It cannot be denied there are differences between them and the London people, yet both groups are welded in unseen bonds of faith—faith in the Almighty, faith in their concepts and faith in themselves as Englishmen. Once we are at sea I firmly believe their mutual disagreements will vanish and give way to fair understanding.

I find myself loath to leave country, home and kin to venture forth to a new domain of which little is known except that it is a merciless, uncivilized land inhabited by wild beasts of the forest and brutish savages called Indians. England's green meadows and heather hedges are exceedingly fair to the eye and never more dear to the heart than at this dismal hour before parting. Yet I must inwardly confess that even dearer is the affection I have taken for the maid Elizabeth, and where the heart draws, there perforce must I follow.

Wednesday, September 6, 1620

We are off on our voyage! Before us lie a thousand leagues or more of unchartered seas. Strong winds and fierce storms lurk in wait to assail our little craft. For weeks and weeks we shall be confined to our narrow, crowded quarters aboard the *Mayflower*, and no doubt sicknesses and diseases will reap a rich harvest among our people. It is not unlikely that the specters of famine and death will stalk us. Who can say? Yet I have a premonition that this time there will be no returning. Either we arrive at America or find our graves in the far-off depths of the sea.

It now appearing that the *Mayflower* will be our home for some time to come, a few words of its housing conditions would not be amiss. We are quartered on the lower deck in two parallel rows of dank and gloomy cabins no bigger than cuddies. They were hastily built to hold not more than one or two in comfort, but we are pressed for room and in each of them there are from three to five people packed in like herrings in pails. Wherever possible the members of one family occupy a cabin by themselves; otherwise the people are thrown together in a makeshift manner. Light and air come in by way of portholes and through the hatchway leading down from the upper deck.

Our material comforts are too mean to be worthy of mention.

The ship's officers are housed in three cabins under the high poop deck at the stern, Captain Jones occupying the largest cabin and his four mates sharing the two smaller ones. The seamen are quartered in the forecastle at the ship's bow on the upper deck. To my mind their abode is of a more favorable situation than ours, mainly by virtue of its higher elevation. It will not be subjected to waves which may sweep the deck and flood our cabins, and they have freer access to light, sunshine and fresh air. All that can be said for our quarters is that we will be better protected against strong winds.

To resume my relation, throughout the day the spirits of the people have been at a low ebb. I had thought our departure would tend to cheer them, but due to the fact that the leave-taking at Plymouth was doleful in the extreme it has proved otherwise. Nor am I better situated than the rest, for I am clutched in the throes of a homesickness exceeding any I have ever known. It is clawing at me with such power that it is all I can do to force myself to record the events which transpired up to this time.

Our Company spent the preceding night aboard the *Mayflower* in readiness for the sailing. Each one whiled away the hours according to his lights, some being wrapped in prayer and meditation while others succumbed to restless slumber. In the main, however, there was a great deal of talk concerning the dangers we were likely to encounter at sea and on our arrival in America. The dangers of the sea are known to all, but our people are not acquainted of their own knowledge with the new land or the customs of its inhabitants.

Neither prayer nor sleep was greatly to my liking, and before the evening was over I crept up to the forecastle to see what could be gleaned in the way of first hand information from the mariners. A group of them had gathered about Tom English, a pox-faced, weatherbeaten old seaman who was relating a passage he had made some two years ago in a ship that went to fish and trade along the coast of New England. He spoke of it as being a goodly land, well wooded and suitable for habitation; but the people there were savages, being cruel and treacherous and most merciless to their enemies.

To judge from his tales of the bloody tortures the Indians inflict on their captives, they cannot be other than a race of fiends. I shuddered as I drank in his gruesome relation. The mariners themselves betrayed their inward quakings by the fearful glances they cast at each other. One of them ventured to inquire if the Indian women were of the same ungentle disposition as their menfolk. I did not linger to hear the discussion likely to follow. The hour was late, and I went back to my cabin.

It was then past midnight and I tumbled into bed to snatch some sleep. An hour or two before daybreak a tumult aroused me from my slumber. I stirred drowsily and listened. Footsteps and voices sounded in the passageway outside my cabin. The people of our Company were trooping forth from their quarters and ascending the hatchway. I awakened my two cabin mates, and after dressing we joined the assemblage on the upper deck.

A dense mist had seeped up from the water, making the early morning air thick and murky, and partly obscuring the view of Plymouth harbor and its environs. The masts and spars of the *Mayflower* loomed gaunt and forlorn above us, and beyond in the distance the moon shone faintly through the haze and was barely visible as its last feeble rays were cast earthward. It was a ghastly scene, made all the more eerie by the fitful glare from lanterns suspended on the deck.

Fretful and impatient, the people paced to and fro, and the Elders clustered about the burly form of Captain Jones who was striving to pierce the fog for weather signs. Streaks of light appeared on the eastern horizon and a light breeze sprang up, dispelling the mist that enveloped us. The skies were clear except for a mass of clouds directly overhead, drifting westward slowly but with increasing speed. After a brief delay Captain Jones ruptured the silence with the glad tidings that the wind was fair and we would sail with the tide within the hour. Our people passed a few moments in joyous congratulations and then went ashore for their leave-taking from many friends and acquaintances.

Plymouth harbor was aclatter and agog with our departure, the *Mayflower* centering all attentions and humming like a beehive in the bustle and confusion of sailing. The quay fairly reeked with townsfolk and spectators who had come swarming down to bear witness to the event. It was a motley throng; friends and foes could be numbered among them as they stood about in parcels and chattered like magpies. Many had come to wish us Godspeed, others to prophesy dark forebodings and some few, alas, to revile us unjustly as 'Brownists' and 'Dissenters' and proclaim England the richer for being rid of us.

This was our third departure from England, yet by far the saddest one. We had found Plymouth a friendly, hospitable town, and its people had done their utmost to extend us every comfort during our sojourn with them. Parting from them was like taking leave from the dearest kin we were never to see again. Also, where before we had sailed with the *Speedwell* for company, we were now setting forth in one lone ship across the vast ocean. Should any mishap befall the *Mayflower*, we would be without hope of human succor or rescue.

Now that the hour to sail was at hand, it was plain that our people were prey to these sober apprehensions and none but were reflecting of the firm-footedness of English soil and the grave uncertainties of this reckless venture. Stern and ashen-hued they said their last farewells, some brokenly and others with quavering voices. Many more could not contain their grief. Strong men gave way and wept beside their more tender womenfolk, and the crying of children served to add fuel to the distraction. Tears flowed freely from all eyes; yea, even our enemies who had come to confound us could not restrain themselves, and so like Balaam they gave us their blessing instead.

As I stood in the midst of these sorrowful displays of love and affection, I became tainted with them and a longing welled up within me to be nigh unto my own kin. Yea, the heart cried aloud and I yearned to be back in the fold wherein I might round out my years in peace and contentment with those loved ones so endeared to me. And thus at the last moment I lost stomach for the venture and wavered in uncertainty as I debated which course to pursue.

It was then that a soft hand reached for mine, and a tender voice, Elizabeth's, said somewhat timidly: "Come, John. The *Mayflower* is ready to sail."

For a brief space the weights trembled in the balance and conflicting emotions surged and ran riot within me. Then the die was cast and we boarded the ship together.

The wind was blowing strongly East North East and we weighed anchor to sail from Plymouth. Heartsick and depressed I retired to my cabin in search of solitude. The wave of homesickness had stirred up emotions which would not be quelled easily, and I preferred to stay below until we had cleared the harbor.

Here I bring to a halt this day's relation, though there are other matters to record. But being downcast and moody, I am not in the temper for it and at present I forbear to say more.

Thursday, September 7, 1620

The sight of land has been lost to the eye since morning. Look where one will, nothing rewards the gaze except the limitless skies and the green-blue expanse of open seas. It is fascinating to observe the countless millions of waves as they rear their white-crested heads and momentarily dance in the sun, only to crumble and fall back into the sea. Countless other millions rise up in their stead, and so it goes on and on without ceasing.

Encompassed by the wonders of nature, serene and omnipotent, it might be thought we mortals would draw sustenance therefrom and rise above the infirmities of our race. Yet how feeble, how frail is mankind! With land less than a day's sail distant, we already are beset with grief and woe; our cup is filled to overflowing. But here I had best resume my relation where I left off yesterday when our miseries had their inception.

By the time we were out of Plymouth harbor I had recovered sufficient composure to warrant my leaving the cabin and going up on deck. Our people were grouped at the starboard with their eyes affixed hungrily to the shore. The *Mayflower*, her full sail trimmed to an overly brisk wind, was racing westward along the coast of Cornwall. Heavy waves from the open sea were surging under her

keel, and she was rolling and tossing like a huge cradle.
The result was that two score of the people were afflicted
with seasickness within an hour.

The first to fall a victim was Edward Thompson, a
servant in the family of William White. It was distracting
to observe how the ailment affected him. He was standing a few paces from me and I heard him remark that he
felt faint. He lurched toward the hatchway, his features
contorted and of a ghastly hue; then he suddenly brought
his hands to his midriff and lumbered to the ship's stern.
With his head distended over the edge he began to retch
and cast up with such violence that I thought his very
entrails would be disgorged into the sea.

Several of us ran to his aid and propped him up while
Dr. Samuel Fuller, our physician, was summoned. He
came bustling through the spectators and took in the
situation at a glance, saying: "It's but an attack of seasickness. No great harm will come of it, I'll warrant.
Come, lads, let's get him below where the pitching of the
ship is not so marked."

We helped Thompson to his cabin and placed him on
his bed. He was in a pitiful condition. The convulsions
had sapped his strength, leaving him in a state of utter
exhaustion. His head hung limply at his breast and his
limbs dangled awkwardly as though he were a poppet.
Particles of the food he had disgorged were coated on the
front part of his clothing, and its savor was most offensive.

Dr. Fuller dissolved a measure of salts in a cup of water

and forced him to drink it to physic his inners. He quaffed it with a wry face and had another convulsion. Soon thereafter he was somewhat relieved, though he continued to moan in agony.

While we were standing about, John Hooke, a servant boy, came dashing in and shouted: "Dr. Fuller, you're wanted on deck. Many of the people have been taken sick."

The physician hastily departed and went clambering helter-skelter up the steps of the hatchway. I followed after him, and on reaching the upper deck I stood amazed at the sight that greeted my eyes. At every side there was nothing to be seen but men, women and children stationed at intervals along the ship's edge and casting up in the same manner as Thompson. Mingled with their groans were the quips and jests of the seamen who seemed in high glee over the miseries of the distressed ones.

I had never borne witness to such a scene of affliction, nor was there time to stand in idle contemplation. There was work to be done, and those of us who were firm afoot rushed to the task of aiding the sickly. Some were so weakened they had fallen prostrate, and these we bore below to their cabins to await the visitation of Dr. Fuller with his never-failing store of salts. Then we aided those whose condition was considered as being of less consequence.

By sundown fully half of our Company had fallen prey to the sickness and our quarters had acquired the earmarks of a pesthouse. In every cabin one or more sick ones tossed in anguish. They groaned unceasingly in their extremities and continued so throughout the night, to the great discomfort of those who were free from the affliction. I lay awake waiting for the hours to spend themselves, and when morning came I thankfully arose and went above to make a survey of our situation.

A huge, red-blood sun was rising out of the sea on the eastern horizon, and to the south of us the sky was fringed with an array of tufted white clouds. The wind had veered during the night to East South East, almost blowing a gale and filling the air with showers of fine spray. Our sails were puffed and bloated outward by its force. The *Mayflower* was flying westward at a rate of speed she had heretofore failed to display.

Not many of our Company were to be encountered on deck, the only ones being John Rigdale, Solomon Prower and John Langermore, all London men. They were at the starboard near the stern, gazing across the sea at the southwestern point of England's shore, known as Land's End.

I sauntered in their direction and tendered them greetings of the day. John Rigdale half turned his head and muttered a response; the other two were silent. I perceived they were in a cheerless humor, yet I essayed a faint-hearted effort to strike up a discourse. They were even more sparse in their speech, and I abandoned any further attempt to draw them from their reticence.

As the morning advanced, others of the people joined us from time to time. They were haggard and worn from lack of sleep and their lackluster appearances were in conformity with their drooping spirits. Some of the children accompanied them, hovering about their listless elders in silent accord. A more dreary and woebegone lot could not be contemplated.

All eyes were glued on Land's End, by this time a faint jot scrawled on the horizon in the far northeast and barely visible to the naked eye. It was even of interest to our sick ones, for word came that many of them were praying to be brought on deck. We aided them up from below, and truly they made a doleful spectacle. Tears coursed down their furrowed cheeks and the womenfolk sobbed gently as they drank their fill of the last view of English soil. Before long it failed to the sight and the final link to the land of our nativity was severed.

This was the last straw. Throughout the day the people were immersed in a pall of gloom and the oncoming night found them at the mercy of dismal thoughts and given over to dull despair. Of a certainty the grief of our departure has left its mark.

Friday, September 8, 1620

Last night I went to bed in a state of dejection and with little hope of slumber. Nor did I err in my judgment, for I was kept awake by the moaning of the sick. Their cries welled up in a tumult resounding through our quarters like the lowing of thirsty kine. Hour after hour it continued without abatement, and though I desperately strove to close my eyes, it was of no avail. Finally at three or four o'clock in the morning I arose and went on deck to await the break of dawn.

A mellow moon was drifting low in the southern sky and cast its beams on the water athwart the larboard bow. The breeze had fallen off somewhat; the sea appeared calm with waves no bigger than ripples on a pond. On deck at the helm I discerned the lone figure of a seaman muffled to the ears to ward off the chill night air. I felt impelled to join him for companionship sake, but I desisted. There is bad blood between the seamen and our people, and I had no relish for the thought of being rebuked by him.

As the night wore on the wind quickened, blowing with greater force, and I sensed the *Mayflower* leaping forward like a steed under the spurs. The waves were whipped into a frenzy, and by morning they came rolling higher than any we had encountered. With the ship heaving and tossing in an unruly manner, I surmised it would be an evil day for the people, and so it proved. They were sorely ravaged by seasickness; at midday the affliction had gained the mastery of all but a scant score of our Company. Dr. Fuller, himself, gave way and is a victim to the malady. Now there is none to aid our distressed and relieve their ills, since the ship's surgeon, Dr. Giles Heale, holds himself aloof from us as not being in his particular charge.

I spent most of the day below tending the sick as best I could and bartering confidences with my two cabin mates, John Alden and Will Butten. John Alden is a cooper we had hired at Southampton. He is a pleasant youth of many graces, tall, broad-shouldered and with flowing yellow hair, and though a smith by trade he gives tongue to fair words and phrases which find a ready welcome in every ear. He is not admitted into fellowship with those of the Leyden Church, nor has he requested communion with them, but thinks to return to England when his time runs out.

Will Butten is serving his apprenticeship under Dr. Fuller. He is a promising lad and a seasoned student of medicine and alchemy. His luggage is cluttered with musty tomes into which he is ever delving deeply to slake his thirst for the learning of these arts. A maid in Austerfield has plighted him her troth, and he will send for her after he has made a home in America.

We sat conversing in an atmosphere reeking with foul odors cast off by the sick and which kept filtering through our quarters. Toward sundown I felt ill from it and started to go on deck for a breath of fresh air. The cabin opposite ours is occupied by Stephen Hopkins, a London man of considerable affluence as is attested by the fact that he has two servants, Edward Dotey and Edward Leister. As I passed by, he hailed me to come in and I entered, finding him with his wife and three children, all in a wretched state of sickness.

"Lad, call Dr. Fuller," he said, heaving and gasping as though drawing his last breath. "This misery is more than I can withstand."

"I will gladly do so, Mr. Hopkins," I answered, "but I doubt if he can come. He's ill himself."

"I know it, but it may be he's recovered. Likely as not he has found a way to mend his own ills while we poor mortals suffer. Go, lad, and make known to him it's urgent."

I left on my mission and returned empty-handed.

"Dr. Fuller is deathly sick," I told him. "He cannot come now, but will do so as soon as he's able. Meanwhile he bids you to hold your patience."

"Patience, patience," fumed Stephen Hopkins, half rising. "Here I lie on what may prove to be my deathbed and he speaks to me of patience. Did one ever hear the like of it before? Is he bereft of reason? Patience indeed."

"Stephen, be calm," pleaded Mrs. Hopkins weakly.

"I'll not be calm," he cried in a heat. "I'll not stand idly by while we all perish on this madcap voyage. Where are the Elders? Why don't they turn back while there's time? Go summon them to me, lad."

I hesitated, and he sat up and glared at me with his pale blue eyes peering through red-rimmed eyelids.

"Why do you linger," he shouted. "Are you rooted to the ground? Now do as I bid you. Go summon the Elders to me at once."

"But Mr. Hopkins," I stammered. "They're all ill."

"Not more so than I am," he replied. "If they'll not come, then I'll order the ship's captain to sail back to port. Tell them what I said, and it's no idle threat either."

He bristled with wrath and I hastily departed to see which of the Elders could be mustered. None of them paid me any heed, nor would they stir from their cabins except my patron, John Carver, whom we consider the foremost man of our Company. He alone accompanied me back to Stephen Hopkins' cabin.

"Why don't we put back to England?" demanded Stephen Hopkins. "The people are sick and there's no hope of succor. Our physician can do nothing for us. Are we to wait till all are dead from their infirmities? I say, let's make sail back to port while there's still life left in us."

"Mr. Hopkins, your affliction has warped your better judgment," said John Carver gently. "The seasickness is not a fatal ailment. In due time and with the Lord's help all will be restored to health. This voyage was undertaken by us in an honorable cause and for a most worthy end. If it should entail some suffering, we must bear it bravely."

Stephen Hopkins was somewhat mollified, yet not wholly quelled. "It's a simple matter for you to talk about enduring pain. You are childless. But consider that I have three little ones. Am I, the father, to see them racked with torture before my eyes and say nothing?"

"There is weight in what you say," answered John Carver. "And truly it grieves me fully as much as it does you to see the little ones in affliction. Yet I repeat they will recover shortly and be none the worse for it. Nay, Mr. Hopkins. We've embarked on this voyage and we'll not face about unless the Lord wills it otherwise."

He bowed his grey head for a moment as though in silent prayer and then withdrew, a somber figure of majesty. Stephen Hopkins fell back on his bed muttering under his breath, and I went on deck.

The wind had lessened its force, though the waves were still pounding the ship's keel with vigor. High up on the masts and spars the seamen were reefing the topsails. On the far western horizon the sun was dipping slowly into the sea. Another day ended, a day nearer our haven. How many more days would pass before we arrived there? And what does fate hold in store for us on our arrival? Thus for a time I mused in solitude and then retired for the night.

Saturday, September 9, 1620

I am weary of sleepless nights and more weary writing of them. This morning I arose with my eyes half closed. John Alden was wrapped in slumber, but Will Butten's bed was unoccupied. It is a matter of great envy to me that John Alden sleeps through these troublesome nights as though nothing were amiss. Will Butten, I suspected, was up and about attending the sickly. Since Dr. Fuller's illness he has filled the breach in an admirable fashion.

On leaving the cabin I was accosted by Mrs. Catherine Carver, John Carver's wife. Of the eighteen wives in our Company she is one of the few who have thus far escaped the affliction of seasickness. Upon her has fallen the burden of preparing sustenance for the sickly, and being childless she has borne the brunt cheerfully. She makes them such victuals as are best suited for their needs. This, for the main part, is either broth or pottage made by boiling chicken with barley or groats and then skimming off the fat before serving.

She asked me to bring her six chickens for the day's fare. When I went down to the hold where our fowl are kept, I was thunderstruck to find them scattered throughout the length and breadth of the place and roaming at large over the cargo. Their coops were empty. Someone had maliciously opened the gratings and set the fowl at liberty. There was no need to think twice. I apprehended that the seamen were undoubtedly at the bottom of this wanton act.

It was only one instance of what has been in progress these past few days. The people have been unmercifully beset by the seamen who have made merry over their ills and seek to vex and play them mischief at every turn. Especially a lusty seaman, Tom Shipley, has hectored them beyond measure and is in constant show of such ill will that all have been cursed by him with vile oaths and execrations. He plots with his fellows how best to irk us and is a scourge, a thorn from whom the Elders pray for deliverance.

Daily the Elders have made complaint of this to Captain Jones who seems to be a fair-minded man, as sea-captains go. On each occasion he swore he would not brook his men to disport themselves to our discomfort and the evil-doers he would punish roundly, even clap them in irons if need be. While these words had brought good cheer, the persecutions did not cease and so nothing came of it.

This latest prank of the seamen was a matter of no little annoyance to me. Determined to secure the allotment requested by Mrs. Carver, I exhausted myself in a fruitless effort to drive the fowl back into their coops. They were as elusive as eels; after a good half hour of endeavor my reward was several handfuls of feathers and a score of bruises and sprains. I then desisted and went to inform John Carver of the happening.

A worried look crept into his somber dark eyes.

"Come with me, lad," he said. "We'll report this outrage to the ship's captain."

Captain Jones was on deck conversing with Robert Coppin, the pilot. Several of the seamen were close at hand, and they pricked up their ears to get wind of the discourse.

"Captain Jones, there's no end to the abuse we suffer from your men," said John Carver. "One of them has freed all our fowl and they run loose in the ship's hold. What do you say to that?"

"Freed all your fowl, you say, Mr. Carver?" asked Captain Jones as though incredulous. He shifted uneasily, cast a glance at the nearby knot of seamen and brazenly remarked: "Why I would say it's a foul tale. What would you say, Mr. Coppin?"

Highly pleased with his quip, Captain Jones roared in mirth, accompanied by the pilot and echoed by the seamen.

"Nay, it's not a jesting matter," remarked John Carver. "We have enough grief without being burdened by thoughtless pranksters. We rely on our fowl to sustain our sick, and now they've escaped us. If any of our people should suffer ill effects because of it, the blame will be yours, Captain Jones."

"Come, come, Mr. Carver," said the captain, awakened to the gravity of the situation. "The fowl are still in the hold and can be caught. Besides, who bears witness that any of my men set them free?"

"We have no witness, but I'll take oath that it was not the doing of our people."

"And I'll take oath that my men are not guilty," Captain Jones stoutly averred. "So we're quits on that score."

"That does not remedy the harm."

"Mr. Carver, I'm worn out by the multitude of your complaints," the captain muttered wearily. "Since we sailed from Plymouth I've heard nothing else from you. And where lies the fault, in God's name? If the truth must be told, it's with your people. They're a waspish lot who don't know how to live at peace with their fellowmen. All know they were harried from England to Holland, and now that the Dutch have driven you out, you seek homes among the savages in America. It may be that you'll find peace there, but I doubt it. My men are law-abiding English subjects who quarrel with none. I'll have them trap your precious fowl for you this once, but mind now, Mr. Carver, no more complaints will I hear from you or yours."

"So be it, Captain Jones," replied John Carver stiffly. "I forbear to answer your unjust charges. Yet if we have righteous cause to complain and you will not hear us, then doubtless the Lord will."

There was an air of grandeur in John Carver's words and bearing that transcended and rendered insignificant the puny aspersions cast on our Company. Captain Jones shrugged his shoulders and the seamen essayed a forced laugh which fell short of its purpose. As John Carver swept by, he failed to acknowledge their presence, not according them as much as a glance. There was scant room for debate. He had clearly won the issue and carried off the honors.

During the forenoon the miseries of the sick wreaked havoc with their spirits. A number more tearfully petitioned the Elders to sail back to England. These were mainly London people, and I was inclined to believe that Stephen Hopkins had brought the weight of his influence into play. But the Elders, themselves sorely afflicted, lent deaf ears to their pleas and exhorted them to seek relief in the Lord.

It was shortly past noonday when the sickness gave evidence of falling away. Stephen Hopkins was one of the first to recover. I chanced to go into his cabin and found him engaged in putting a fire under the cooking pot.

"Ha, lad," he exclaimed on seeing me. "I'm well again. My stomach has returned and I hunger for victuals."

"I'm well pleased to hear it, Mr. Hopkins," I replied. "Shall I bring you some broth from Mrs. Carver?"

"Broth? Faugh." He spat his disgust. "I'm fair famished, I could devour an ox from his tail to his horns. For three days I've supped on miserly broth and now I'll dine in state. Go fetch me a chicken, lad. And mind, now, none of your scrawny roosters. Bring me a good fat hen."

I went to the hold on my errand. The fowl had been cooped up again, though to judge from the feathers scattered about, it must have been a worthy tussle for the seamen. I picked out a hen and bore it squawking down the passageway.

As I passed Dr. Fuller's cabin he hailed me and called: "Whom is it for, lad?"

"For Mr. Hopkins," I replied. "He's back to health and almost famished from hunger."

"Say that I warn him not to eat a gross meal," said Dr. Fuller. "He'd best forbear to eat meat for a day or two till he's more fully recovered."

This caution I repeated to Stephen Hopkins, but his hunger was such that he would not be ruled by it.

"Tut, tut," he scoffed as he seized the hen and wrung its neck. "Am I to listen again to Dr. Fuller's nonsense? When I was near death's door yesterday, he bade me to hold my patience. And now that I'm better, no thanks to him, he tells me to starve for my health's sake. A likely physician indeed. Here, Bess," he said to his wife. "Prepare the chicken for the pot. I'll dine on it though the king's own surgeon came and said me 'Nay'."

The pot was soon simmering briskly on the fire and I lingered in the hope that a wing or part of the breast would be awarded me. As the savory, delectable odor was wafted in the air Stephen Hopkins could hardly contain his impatience. He danced about in a heathenish sort of rite, sniffed the vapors and licked his chops in ecstasy.

Every now and then he would raise the lid from the pot to test the tenderness of the meat, though in so doing he delayed the cooking.

When the fowl was done he ripped it into halves and devoured it to the last shred, even crunching some of the smaller bones between his teeth. I was astounded at his gluttony no less than I was vexed at his greed in failing to offer me a slight portion of the repast. Yet even as I turned to leave crestfallen, he paid the penalty for his rashness. He became sick again, being seized with violent retchings and cast up the victuals. I had no sympathy to spare and left him groaning in agony.

A number more were restored to health by nightfall. The disaster that had overtaken Stephen Hopkins stood them in good stead, for they heeded Dr. Fuller and abstained from eating heartily. With the sickness abating, the malcontents are silenced and the morrow gives promise of being a fairer day for us.

Sunday, September 10, 1620

This was our first Sabbath Day at sea and it brought a measure of cheer to dispel our grief and woe. The sickness commenced to disperse in earnest and the weather was the fairest we had encountered since our departure from Plymouth. A gentle wind blowing from the southeast sufficed to fill our sail, yet the sea was calm and unruffled. The *Mayflower* kept on an even keel as she glided steadily over the water like a huge bird on the wing.

Early in the morning I called for Elizabeth and we came on deck together. A goodly number of the people were already assembled there, and considering that many had been confined below these past few days, it was a priceless boon for them to be out in the fresh air. They were visibly wan and pinched, though they had bravely tried to cloak their wasted appearances by coming attired in their finest holiday array. With their clothing washed and features cleansed to the bone, they shone like the scrubbed bricks of a newly scoured courtyard.

We were augmented by others of the Company who came up to join with us. It was a joyous congregation. Greetings of the day passed back and forth, solicitous inquiries were directed concerning the health of each and the discourse was free and affable. Under these auspicious influences the withered spirits of the people blossomed anew and soared skyward. I had never seen so complete a change in men and women in so brief a span of time.

We were guided in prayer by the Ruling Elder, William Brewster, a venerable, white-bearded man of godly mien and tender heart. Having no pastor of their own, the London people found themselves in an awkward situation at the start of the services. Some few joined in with us. These included William Mullins, his wife and daughter Priscilla, Edward Fuller and his wife, Richard Warren and Gilbert Winslow. The rest hung back in a body within earshot and yet at a distance. Evidently they wanted some leeway that might enable them to refute the charge of heresy if it ever should be lodged against them.

Elder Brewster preached an eloquent sermon wherein he exhorted us to make a humble and open confession of sin and then concluded the services with a benediction. Like a prophet of old he stood in our midst with his eyes closed and his hands raised aloft as he called down the Lord's blessing on us and compassionately beseeched His forgiveness for our transgressions.

It was a brave sight to the eye with the azure sky above, sails taut in the wind, the swirl of the sea below, and on deck our people pouring out their hearts in fervent prayer and making melody in the singing of psalms to His glory.

What evil has come upon me? My head has turned giddy and the entrails rise within me as if to disgorge themselves. I can write no more.

Thursday, September 14, 1620

For three days I tossed in my cabin and moaned in the extremities of the seasickness that came upon me last Sunday night. Of a certainty it is without a peer among the afflictions to which mankind is subjected. The head aches as though it were being rent asunder, the world sways dizzily before one's eyes, the entrails stubbornly deny ingress to victuals and the body is racked with successive fits of convulsion.

I lay in torment with all conception of time lost to me. Day and night were alike, each hour was akin to the one last past. Nor was it physical anguish alone that I suffered. It provoked me to think that a sound, robust body like mine should give way to the illness while others, more feeble than I, could withstand its attack. I was aware that Dr. Fuller forced vile concoctions down my throat and Elizabeth was ever hovering at my bedside. Several times I prayed for her to leave me and I would take joy in dying rather than endure the miseries that beset me.

However, I will not dwell overlong on the tortures of my confinement. This morning, praised be the Lord, the ailment has flown, and I pray it may never return. I was aided from my musty cabin up to the deck. In the warm sun and the brisk salty air, I marveled that I now held

death so little to my liking and the love of life so dear.
So it is with mankind. At a time of stress we clamor to
look death in the face and extend it open arms, yet when
the ordeal is over we soundly berate ourselves for having
done so.

The people came pressing about me with kind words
and unfeigned expressions of hope for my quick recovery.
I learned that nothing noteworthy had occurred aboard
ship during my illness. I had been one of the last to be
afflicted with seasickness. Some half a score were still dis-
abled, but it was thought the week's end would see them
all restored to health.

It was cool and pleasant on deck, but as noonday approached the breeze died off and the sun waxed exceedingly hot as it ascended overhead. I was forced to go
below to my cabin to seek relief, and feeling drowsy I lay
on my bed and fell asleep.

Some time later I was awakened by nearby voices
raised in anger. An altercation was in progress outside my
cabin door. The disputants I recognized as Stephen Hopkins and Isaac Allerton, one of the Leyden Elders.

"And by whose orders are the fowl kept under lock and
key?" Stephen Hopkins turbulently demanded.

"The Elders have decreed it," answered Isaac Allerton.

"Indeed! Then I'll thank you to give me the key for a
moment," said Stephen Hopkins.

"For what purpose?"

"Need I state my purpose?" he roared. "Need I account to you for my each and every act and deed? This is a pretty state of affairs. If you must know, Mr. Allerton, I'm moved to compassion for the fowl and would pluck the lice from them before they're bitten to death. Now you know my purpose, and if you've observed how the poor fowl teem with vermin you'll agree it's a worthy one."

"Such levity is unbecoming you, Mr. Hopkins."

"And such interrogations are unbecoming to you when they're addressed to me," retorted Stephen Hopkins. "What am I, a stripling, that I need run to you and ask, 'Mr. Allerton, may I do thus, and Mr. Allerton, may I do so?' Go to, and do not cross me. I'm not the man to be balked by you or anyone else, for that matter."

At this point I heard John Carver break in to inquire: "Why are you wrangling?"

"He demands the key to the storeroom where the fowl are kept," explained Isaac Allerton. "But he will not state for what purpose."

"What is your reason for wanting the key?" asked John Carver.

"Reason enough. I would have a chicken for my family's dinner," Stephen Hopkins admitted.

"Nay, it cannot be," said John Carver. "Our store of fowl is running low and none will be left for breeding if we continue to consume them. The Elders have ordained that the fowl are to be conserved, except as food for the sickly. Your family is back to health, Mr. Hopkins, and your wife and little ones as well as yourself can dine on simpler fare."

"The Elders decree this and the Elders ordain that," he bellowed in rage. "Who are the Elders and who chose them to be our overlords that they ride over us roughshod and refuse us our least desires? I know full well that you of Leyden are leagued in conspiracy against us of London. You keep us in restraint as though we are your bond-slaves and you our masters. You deny yourselves nothing and partake of the best. Out of sweet charity's sake you throw us a crust of dry bread every now and then as you would a bone to a dog. The London people are aflamed, they cry out daily. You had best tread softly, Mr. Carver. You're creating a schism in our Company, I warn you."

"You know well there is no truth in your slanderous statements," answered John Carver. "If we are to become a body politic then every man must repress his own convenience when it conflicts with the common welfare. Otherwise it would bring us all to ruin. Nor have we shown favor to the Leyden people more so than disfavor to those from London. All are alike in our eyes even as they are in the eyes of the Lord. If any have been unjustly treated, let them seek redress and they shall have it."

John Carver paused to lend effect to his words and then continued in a conciliatory tone. "Now it may be that you have unwittingly received a small slight, Mr. Hopkins, and to make amends you can have a fowl this once. However, we can spare a rooster better than a hen."

"Why not a hen," he grumbled. "A rooster's tough flesh would make poor eating for my children."

"Let it be a hen," agreed John Carver.

The discourse ceased and the footsteps died away. Though it undoubtedly was prudent to let Stephen Hopkins gain his point as a peace offering, I was loath to see it. It will be a feather in his cap and he is certain to preen it to best advantage. He has shown himself to be an arrogant, self-willed man and is one of the chief of the London people.

True, as he stated, there is a schism between them and our Leyden people, but not through any fault of the latter. The Londoners in the main are uncouth and tend to be dissolute, holding those from Leyden in ridicule as being too stiff-necked. The Leyden people on their part are somewhat aghast at the shortcomings of the Londoners, yet they hold the tongue close to the cheek.

Nor is the rift in our Company of recent date. It had its inception soon after those from Leyden arrived in the *Speedwell* at Southampton and there found the London people awaiting them in the *Mayflower*. First they had fallen to joyful greetings and then to bitter wrangling, continuing so to this time. I shall not retrace the unhappy details; the least said the better. But it is evident they still rankle and fester new sores. If further dissension should ensue, it will prove a stumbling-block in our path. A house divided cannot stand.

Friday, September 15, 1620

The weather holds fair and the number of our sick is now whittled down to a handful. Despite an occasional flare of discord such as occurred yesterday, life aboard ship would be passable and even pleasant if it were not for the people being constantly harassed by the seamen. There is no relief from them. They are as evil and degenerate a crew as was ever assembled on one deck.

Due to the known perils of the voyage Captain Jones had been hard pressed to secure seamen who would sail with him. The most thumbed their noses despite the lure of higher wages, and he was well content to hire such as presented themselves without too close a scrutiny of their moral qualities. It is no marvel, then, that they were perforce combed from the wharves among the cast-offs and comprise some of the worst of seafarers, a class that is none too good even at its best.

I do not seek to heap unwarranted reproaches on the heads of those who sail before the mast. The sea is a stern, unrelenting taskmaster, and their lot is hard and their calling a most precarious one. Many of them, as is the custom, are bound out as cabin boys while still in their tender years. They are cast in with older seamen who possess a multitude of vices and few virtues worthy of the name. The vices they readily acquire, the virtues are generally discarded by the wayside with their own. Before long they are shorn of godliness, their spirits are broken under the lash and they become little better than beasts in human form.

It may be that the seamen of the *Mayflower* are no worse than the rest of their ilk, but of a certainty they are no better. One and all they take a fiendish delight in tormenting us, following the leadership and in the footsteps of the fellow Tom Shipley whom I have already mentioned. He is choked with venom like a serpent and will not cease abusing the people. He tells them they are weaklings and starvelings, and before we come to haven it would not grieve him a whit to cast their bodies into the sea to be food for the fishes tarrying in the ship's wake.

This day in the forenoon an incident occurred which aroused my anger to white heat. Two of the Elders, John Carver and William Brewster, accosted Shipley on deck and chided him lightly for his misbehaviors.

"Why do you abuse the people?" asked John Carver. "They've done you no harm, yet you harry them and will not leave them in peace. I pray you, refrain from your evil conduct and seek to guide yourself by a better course."

In answer thereto the surly lout let fly a flood of abuse that all but swept them off their feet. They stood dumfounded at his outburst, and he continued to curse them bitterly. Yea, aged and reverend men that they are, he called them 'doddering old greybeards' and viler names, shouting they had best look to their own affairs and be on their way or he would inflict bodily harm on them.

His rage was such that he fairly frothed at the mouth. Indeed I believe he would have put his threat into execution, had he not been restrained by some of his fellows. Two of them were Tom English and John Allerton, seamen who were hired by us and are considered as being in our service rather than Captain Jones'. They soothed Shipley's ire and called him away to game with them.

The Elders did not flinch before him. They held their ground, not fearing his expected onslaught, but prepared to fend him off as they would a mad dog. And truly it warmed the heart to see their display of courage. How like the spirit pervading the Leyden people! In one hand they bear the Lord's Book and in the other a sword ready to be unsheathed at a moment's notice. They seek peace with mankind, asking only that they may be suffered to worship the Almighty as they deem proper. Yet they will not be trampled underfoot without rising in just defense of their precepts.

I was highly incensed with Shipley's misconduct and brooded over it throughout the day to the exclusion of all else. He will be a hard nut to crack. If Captain Myles Standish were in good health, he would not suffer that affairs have come to so sorry a pass with the fellow. Neither would I, for that matter, had not the sickness sapped the vigor from my limbs. When I have fully recovered, it may be I shall buckle with the Philistine.

I have yet another bone to pick with him. Lately I have had a suspicion he casts a covetous eye at Elizabeth. He had best look to himself.

Saturday, September 16, 1620

The issue with Tom Shipley draws rapidly to a head. His heart abounds in malice and he is bereft of all mercy and compassion. Emboldened by the manner in which he rebuffed the Elders yesterday, he now insults the people with the utmost scorn and contempt. They are in such mortal dread of him that none but quake as if seized with an ague at the first sound of his footfall. There seemingly is no relief from his malignant persecution.

So far as they were able, the people evaded him by staying below. Those who went on deck when he was in the vicinage did so at the peril of subjecting themselves to his gross indignities. Past midday, Edward Dotey, one of Stephen Hopkins' servants, came down from the deck with his clothing in disarray and his features bruised. He forthwith complained to his master that Shipley had assaulted him without provocation.

Having a true Englishman's instinct to rise in defense of his retainer, Stephen Hopkins turned livid with rage and cried: "What, he assaulted you, Ned? I'll grind him to chaff-wheat, I'll fill his sides with cold steel. Ha, Bess," he said to his wife. "Where's my sword, quick. I'll settle the score with Shipley once and for all."

Mrs. Hopkins fluttered like a gawky hen as she searched

for the weapon, and he pranced about champing at her delay.

"Stephen, do not go, I pray you," she moaned. "You're a father to three children with another one soon to arrive. What will become of us if something should happen to you?"

"Nothing will happen to me," he answered lightly. "I'll teach the rascal not to meddle with me or mine. I'll thrash him soundly, I'll tan his hide with the flat of my sword. Never fear for me, Bess. I'll return as speedily as I'm done with him."

I do not know what the outcome would have been, but it fell short of performance. He darted out of the cabin, brandishing his weapon and predicting disaster for Shipley. In the passageway he encountered John Carver who stared at him in amazement and asked: "Where are you bound with your sword in hand, Mr. Hopkins?"

"I'm bent on awarding Shipley a proper chastisement," he answered. "It's his rightful due. He's assaulted my servant Ned Dotey, and I'm not the man to brook it. Stand aside and let me pass."

"Nay, think well before you act rashly," urged John Carver. "We cannot countenance any affrays with the seamen. It would do us far more harm than good. If you are hurt, the loss is ours; if he should be injured then his fellows will seek vengeance and all of us will suffer the brunt of their fury. Above all let us avoid needless bloodshed. It will create a feud between them and us, and no one knows where it may lead. Consider my words well, Mr. Hopkins. If they bear the weight of reason, then pocket your injured pride and restrain yourself from doing us a mischief."

Mrs. Hopkins came running to augment John Carver's calmer judgment with her own tearful pleas. Stephen Hopkins wavered and reluctantly admitted: "There is truth in what you say, Mr. Carver. Yet how are we to cope with this offspring of the devil? Who will defend the people from his insults and abuses?"

"You forget, Mr. Hopkins, the Lord will look after His own."

John Carver reverently bowed his head and Stephen Hopkins did likewise. That was the end of it.

I felt in accord with Stephen Hopkins despite the judicious appeal by John Carver. Shall we await the coming of a miracle to deliver us from bondage to the demon Shipley? I for one cannot put up much longer with his lording it over us as if we were less than the dust beneath his feet. He fully outweighs me by thirty pounds, yet even as I write my blood is afire and the speeded pulse forwarns me that I may not be able to avoid coming to grips with him. Yet I will endeavor to keep John Carver's words in mind.

Before closing my relation for this day I had best mention a matter of a more pleasing nature which I have been lax in recording. On a tedious voyage such as ours, it is engrossing to note how an affair of the heart has its inception. A seed is sown and takes firm root in fertile soil. It is nourished and flourishes, bit by bit, till it bursts into bloom at some distant date.

Thus I have been observing that the maid Priscilla Mullins is strongly taken with my cabin mate, John Alden. She is ever in his tow like the calf after the cow and dotes over his words as if they were pearls of wisdom from the lips of a sage. And he, for all his pretense of great annoyance because of her attention, is not ill pleased with it. To my mind she has also found favor in his eyes, and it may be that when his time runs out he may have good and weighty cause to stay with us.

Yea, and for a like good and weighty cause have I essayed this perilous venture, and more, even to the world's end if need be.

Sunday, September 17, 1620

This was our second Sabbath aboard ship, and it broke clear and fair with a moderately brisk breeze blowing East South East. The morning air was fragrant with the breath of the sea like the scent of lilacs in bloom. An idle drone pervaded the atmosphere and all was peace and contentment aboard the *Mayflower* as befitted the Lord's Day. All too soon it was to be ruptured by the violence of mortal strife and combat.

The Leyden people came out in force for the prayer services held on deck. Elizabeth wore a grey dress with a cape thrown over the shoulders, and her head was covered by a snug purple bonnet fringed with white at the edges. All the womenfolk were similarly attired, yet it seemed to enhance her loveliness above the others. A few unruly wisps of hair strayed from shelter to play in the wind. She was a vision of purity and as fair a sight as a man could wish to gaze on.

When prayer was ended I walked the deck with her, and we were so engrossed in each other that I gave scant heed to a knot of seamen at the bow. When we came within a few feet I first detected them with Tom Shipley in their midst. Here the voice of prudence whispered we had best turn back, but not wishing to appear a craven in her eyes I rashly flung caution to the winds and we proceeded onward.

As we drew abreast of them Shipley sprang out, seized Elizabeth and drew her to him, saying: "Have you a kiss to spare for me, my pretty maid?"

She shrieked aloud and struggled in his arms while the seamen laughed and made merry with coarse jests at her distraction.

For a moment I was spellbound and powerless. Then I knew the time had come to balance our accounts, and I leaped at his throat like a mastiff to throttle him. He loosened his grip on Elizabeth and without further ado he and I joined issue, dealing lusty blows and buffets and thwacking each other with right good will. The seamen encircled us instantly, for a brawl is precious dear to their hearts, and gave vent to joyous shouts as they egged on their fellow to shred my limbs.

The furor was great and threw the ship into an uproar. Many of our people hastened to witness the scuffle, all atremble for my safety and lending me no encouragement with the voice, but rather in silent prayer to the Lord to come to my aid. And their prayers were answered. Such was the desperate fury of my attack that Shipley, who was but a bully at heart, gave ground to my advance and was sorely pressed by me. He then looked to his familiars for succor and two seamen advanced like snarling wolves from the pack to do me mischief.

Now it would have fared ill with me, when lo! Into the

circle strode Captain Standish whom I had thought to be sick abed. And what a figure he cut with his flaming red beard! He was barefooted; his nightshirt protruded above the waist and below it was tucked inside his unbelted breeches. With his left hand he sustained his breeches and in his right hand was leveled a snaphance. To complete the incongruous vision, a nightcap was awry on his head.

He quickly confronted the two seamen and swore an outlandish Dutch oath. They halted in discomfort and he gruffly warned them they had best stand back, for he would brook no foul play and would pistol the first to move a step forward. Forthwith the seamen turned tail and slunk off like curs under the lash.

His hope of succor dispelled by this strange means, Shipley's courage shrunk to nothing. He offered but feeble resistance and I assailed him with such renewed vigor that the outcome was not long left in doubt. A shrewd buffet cast him headlong and he cried quits, craving mercy of me. But alas. Where had flown the meek spirit of Christian love and forgiveness? All gentle and tender I aided him upright and then struck him a fearful clout for good measure, leaving him sprawled on deck to wallow in his gore.

The conflict was over and I stood in a daze, conscious that shouts of 'huzza!' were resounding in my ears. Accompanied by a hearty thump on my back, Captain Standish said: "Well done, lad, well done indeed. I'll warrant

the fellow will not venture to cross swords with you again.
But that last blow you dealt him— Ha! That was a master
stroke. It was worth a pretty penny to see."

I made light of it, though I was well pleased with his
words, and mumbled my thanks for his having warded off
the seamen.

"That was nothing," he replied. "The swine hardly
know the meaning of fair play. I wish they had come
forward. It would have done me good to dispatch both.
But hearken, lad— It was the maid Elizabeth who came
to summon me. She has your welfare at heart, perhaps
even more. Do you know it?"

I felt myself getting red as I stammered in an effort to
reply evasively.

"So that's how the rooster crows," he cried, breaking
into laughter. "Good enough then. You'd best go and
have your wounds dressed. You've done yourself proud
for the day."

I withdrew to my cabin, trailed by loud applause from
the people. The Elders, I thought, eyed me in stony
silence, and I was somewhat disturbed by their demeanor.
Yesterday's discourse between John Carver and Stephen
Hopkins had slipped from my mind in the heat of battle,
but I now recalled it with pin-prickings of the conscience.
Yet I could not see where I had been at fault and waved
my qualms away.

I had not emerged scathless from the affray. I was a
sight to behold. My battered, bloody features bore ample

evidence to the impact of Shipley's blows and my clothing had been ripped to shreds, hanging piecemeal from my back. Every bone and muscle groaned in agony as if I had been drawn through a mangle. Yet when Elizabeth came to help Dr. Fuller bathe my wounds, I felt fully compensated for my aches and pains.

Monday, September 18, 1620

My bout with Shipley brought me glory of no small measure and a surprising aftermath. I had nursed my bruises and swollen joints before sheer physical exhaustion had closed my eyes in slumber. Toward daybreak I was aroused by a thumping on the door. Will Butten opened it and in came Stephen Hopkins, Edward Dotey, Edward Leister and two other Londoners, crowding the cabin to the hilt.

"Good morning, lad. We've come to crown you with the laurels you've won for yourself," said Stephen Hopkins, waxing eloquent. "It was a worthy deed and we're indebted to you with our utmost gratitude. I speak for all of us, do I not?"

The others chorused in agreement, and Edward Dotey said: "He smote the son of Anak, hip and thigh."

"Well said, Ned, well said, though you've filched the words from my tongue, you rascal. It ill becomes you to be so forward before your master." Stephen Hopkins frowned and then, not to be outdone, added: "But I'll drive it a notch higher. Here and now I'll maintain against all odds that the lad was the instrument of the Lord and smote the Philistine even as David smote Goliath. What do you say to that?"

His words evoked another chorus of approval which caused him to brighten perceptively. By this time I was sufficiently awakened to voice my protest at their homage.

"Tut, tut, lad," said Stephen Hopkins. "We give you no more than is your rightful due. Modesty is a becoming virtue if not carried to excess, so do not seek to belittle your accomplishment. I, myself, would have done it had I not been held in abeyance by Mr. Carver, plague take him for it. There I was itching to slice Shipley as I would a leg of mutton, and the old simpleton waylays me with soft words and steers me from my avowed purpose."

"You would have done it as well as I, Mr. Hopkins," I said.

"That may be," he answered regretfully. "But the fact remains that while I *might* have done it, you're the one who *did* do it. You've earned the esteem of our entire Company and gained a firmer friend in Stephen Hopkins. I like your mettle, lad. If you're ever in need of me, I'm at your command."

The others expressed themselves in a similar vein. I thanked them for their proffers and they took their leave. That was only the prologue. The entire morning I was beset with people who came to gloss with me and puff my victory. At first modesty forbade me to heed their praise, yet in the end I lent a ready ear and even hungered for it. Thus humility was cast out and vanity firmly enthroned in its place. For the time I was cock of the walk.

But alas, how pride foreruns the fall. At noonday Will

Latham, a servant lad, came to inform me that John
Carver requested my presence. I was filled with misgivings on hearing this; then, being flushed with self-esteem,
I bolstered myself with the presumption that I was summoned to be extended further honors.

At John Carver's cabin, I found him with the chief
men of our Company: William Brewster, William Bradford, Isaac Allerton and Edward Winslow, all gathered
in solemn assemblage. I looked in vain for Dr. Fuller who
is also accounted among our leaders, and from his absence I inferred the council had been called to censure,
not praise me.

Nor was I long left in doubt about the matter. Without
delay John Carver, the spokesman, denounced me
openly, saying: "You stand before us charged with sundry acts committed contrary to the peace and dignity of
our Church, and you must answer for them. You have
profaned the Lord's Day by a needless act of violence,
you have shed blood in lusty combat, you have breached
the peace in the sight of the multitude, you have taken
vengeance out of the Lord's hand into your own. Now
what have you to say in answer?"

I stood muted in awe, overwhelmed by the enormity of
my sins, and could make no reply.

"By his silence he confesses his guilt," announced John
Carver.

They are grave and reverend men, the Elders, shep-
herds of the flock, and each in turn chided me for my

misdeeds, not harshly but sternly in reproof. Having concluded they bowed their heads in prayer and Elder Brewster pleaded for the Lord to forgive me my transgressions
and lead me in the path of righteousness.

Fallen am I from grace and humbled in the dust.

Tuesday, September 19, 1620

The news of my chastisement has filtered through the Company. Captain Standish fumed and Stephen Hopkins fretted. Others came with whispered words of encouragement out of earshot of the Elders. But it is to no avail. My heart is weighted as if with lead and I cannot hold my head up for shame. What more need be said?

Wednesday, September 20, 1620

A fortnight has elapsed; yea, fourteen days ago the *Mayflower* sailed from Plymouth. Thus far the Lord in His infinite mercy has blessed the passage with fair weather and prosperous winds, and the people are mightily encouraged by reason of being healed of their sicknesses. A quarter and more of the way is over and Captain Jones avers if all goes well a month to five weeks at the most will see us secure in haven. Yet in the face of this I am forced to write of that which brings no joy to the heart, but only grief and distraction.

I do not sit in at the councils of the Elders. What transpires at their meetings is unbeknown to me as it is to most of the Company. Now and then a word is dropped or a rumor drifts out and passes from tongue to ear as it runs the gantlet through our ranks. These are mere hearsays and deserving of no credence, yet there are other matters of grave concern which are known to all in common. The schism between the Londoners and the Leyden people is one, and another is the cause of the wrangling between the Elders and Christopher Martin, the Treasurer of the Company.

He came from Essex, being one of the people from sundry parts of England who joined with us at Southampton. When negotiations were opened with Thomas Weston's friends, the Adventurers, two agents were sent from Leyden to England to buy provisions for the voyage. At the same time and to avoid any complaints of partiality by the London people, Christopher Martin was chosen from among them to act also as agent and aid the two from Leyden.

As it turned out he proved more a hindrance than a help to them. He was intrusted with £700 at Southampton and spent it in so reckless a manner that he cannot or will not account for it. This has been a bone of contention since our departure. Whenever the Elders ask him for an accounting he flies into a rage and will not answer. To all their pleas and entreaties he turns a deaf ear, and they are at their wits' end and do not know what will come of it.

During the time while the people were burdened with sickness the Elders did not press the matter too strongly, but today in the forenoon it flared up in a violent disputation. John Carver and William Bradford went to Christopher Martin's cabin and again demanded an accounting from him. His voice could be heard in the passageway as he shouted: "You are thankless ingrates. For all my cares and pains I do not merit your suspicions. I'm not beholden to you for an accounting and I'll not give you any except at the proper time. I'll take no more abuse from you Leyden bloodsuckers, and that's an end to it. Now out of my cabin with both of you."

He flung the door open and appeared burning with fury. A group of spectators hastened to the scene, among them Stephen Hopkins who set his corpulent figure into the thick of the fray.

"Speak softly, Mr. Martin," said John Carver as he came out followed by William Bradford.

"I have no need for soft speech," thundered Christopher Martin. "Thieves who come in the night speak in whispers, but honest men don't fear to trumpet their presence."

"Might I ask what's amiss here?" interposed Stephen Hopkins.

"He will not account for the money he spent at Southampton," explained William Bradford.

"It's not the truth," exclaimed Christopher Martin. "I'll give an accounting, but only at the proper time and to the proper authorities. Who are you that you come as magistrates to condemn me for an infamous crime I never committed? Am I to be sentenced without a fair hearing?"

"His words ring with justice," declared Stephen Hopkins, addressing John Carver and William Bradford. "In good truth, who are you that you come bloated with self-appointed powers to accuse an innocent man of wrongdoing? Christopher Martin is an honorable man; he's a stranger to the ways of knavery, I'll warrant. Furthermore I dare say he'll account to our satisfaction when the time is ripe and after we've chosen men in authority who know how to exercise their office without unjust abuses. Do I speak for you, Mr. Martin?"

He nodded vigorously.

"And one thing more, Mr. Carver," continued Stephen Hopkins darkly. "I have a strong suspicion that you persecute Christopher Martin simply for the reason that he's not one of your Leyden people. I know well of what I am speaking. You foster dissension among us faster than I can heal it. The London people will not put up with it much longer. You had best be wary before it's too late."

With this parting shot Stephen Hopkins walked off, paying no heed to a vehement protest by John Carver. The people dispersed talking in undertones, some for and others against Christopher Martin. For my part I do not know what to make of it. He impresses me as an honorable man, though heady and overbearing. No doubt he will render a faithful account in due time, but meanwhile he subjects himself to suspicion and the Company to discord.*

---

* Historical Note: Christopher Martin gave a confused and incomplete accounting when he was on his deathbed at Plymouth, New England, the following January 6th.

Thursday, September 21, 1620

Trouble never comes without being followed by its
consort, and so on the heels of yesterday's occurrence I
have a most grievous relation to make for today. It concerns itself with John Billington who is not of the Leyden
Church, but came from London well-spoken by misguided friends of ours. He is a profane man of vile speech
and unseemly demeanor. Not a day passes but he is in his
cups carousing with the seamen and assailing the Company with ribald talk and song.

How he got his drink was a perplexity to us. Several
times during his absence his cabin was searched for a
hidden supply without the discovery of a single drop.
Notwithstanding this he seemed to have a bounteous
source to tap that more than sufficed for his own needs
and those of his boon drinking companions; yet none
knew where it was or from where it came.

The secret came to light this morning and brought dire
consequences to one of the Company. Isaac Allerton
chanced to go to the storeroom in the ship's hold where
our strong water and spirits are kept under lock and key.
The door was ajar and in the room he trapped John
Billington who had evidently found it a small matter for
one of his thievish talents to pick the lock and gain ad-

mittance. He was drinking his fill from a bottle of spirits as Isaac Allerton entered.

Thus nipped in the bud, Billington uttered a cry like an enraged animal and struck the Elder on the head with the bottle, inflicting a grievous wound. He swooned on the spot and his dastardly assailant fled from the scene to take refuge with the seamen.

Through the Lord's great mercy Isaac Allerton was discovered shortly thereafter or else he surely would have perished from loss of blood. And indeed he was borne to his cabin as one whom we thought dead. His scalp had been laid open to the depth of a finger's width and the life stream seeped out in a steady flow. Dr. Fuller was hard put to stanch it, but after this was accomplished his heart began to beat somewhat stronger.

Seeing her husband brought to this doleful state, Mrs. Allerton had uttered a piercing shriek and fallen in a merciful swoon. She was revived, and the wailing that broke from her and their three children was pitiful to hear. For two hours Isaac Allerton hovered near death with his life barely hanging by a spider's thread. His sight finally came to him, and Dr. Fuller administered a potent draft which helped restore him more fully to consciousness. In a feeble tone he related his encounter with Billington and then fell back exhausted.

The people were wroth beyond measure and the hue and cry was raised to find the culprit and punish him. Our search proved fruitless; look where we would Billington was not to be found. Captain Jones was appealed to, and on being informed of the happening he ordered his men to produce the body of Billington forthwith. The miscreant was uncovered in a recess of the forecastle where he had scurried for shelter and was dragged before the Elders.

"Foul, wretched man," cried John Carver. "See where your evil ways have led you. You struck an innocent, defenseless man with intent to murder him. To escape detection you would have sealed the lips of the witness to your transgression. The enormity of your crime surpasses all bounds; no punishment would be too severe for you. If Isaac Allerton should die, his death will be charged against you. Have you anything to say in your own defense?"

"He came spying on me," whined Billington with a half-defiant air.

"Spying on you, was he?" roared Captain Standish reaching for his sword. "Give me leave to run him through, let me spit him on my sword."

He strained fiercely like a hound on the leash and we had much ado to hold him in restraint.

Billington dropped his defiant pose and fell groveling on the deck. "Have mercy, my masters," he sniveled. "I'm a sickly man and needed the spirits to allay my malady. I did not strike him of my own free will. An evil spirit came into me and caused the bottle to fly from my hand. I tried to hold it back, but some invisible force tore

71

it from my grasp. The deed was not of my own doing, I swear it. Have mercy on me, I pray you."

He rambled on in this vein with great fervency, but his talk was held in small esteem. A discussion ensued as to what should be done with him. Here the Elders were in a quandary. Some said he should be given the lash and others favored searing him with a hot iron. Billington writhed and shrieked in anticipation of the torture, pleading in an anguished voice for them to be merciful to him, a repentant sinner.

Captain Jones was asked for his opinion and gave a terse reply: "String him up on the yardarm."

The Elders recoiled from this suggestion, and counter to it the ever compassionate William Brewster pleaded that Billington be confined for a time on bread and water to expiate his crime and await the outcome of Isaac Allerton's wound. Many demurred, holding it too light a sentence, yet Elder Brewster with his benevolent pleading swayed them to his view. It was so decided. As the cringing villain was led off, he at least had the good grace to give thanks to his benefactor.

William Brewster failed to respond, but William Bradford said: "Mark the words, John Billington. You shall come to an untimely end, and if I'm not mistaken I will live to see you swing from the gallows."*

---

* Historical Note: While William Bradford served as governor of Plymouth, John Billington was brought to trial for the murder of John Newcomen and was hanged for this crime in October, 1630.

Friday, September 22, 1620

When the angel of the Lord has passed by, the devil again puts forth his head. So it is now with Tom Shipley. He has gained ear of the rebuke meted me by the Elders, and made secure thereby he has returned to his last. Not in the open but underhandedly he plays us mischief, fostering hurts and hindrances by the score and going beyond himself to contrive ways and means to vex us. Thanks to him life is voided of joy and the voyage is as full of troubles as a mongrel dog with fleas.

Captain Jones and his mates blink their eyes at his misdeeds; the seamen join in his plots and hearken to his pranks with blasts of mirth resounding like gusts of the north wind. And what can I do but stamp in the stall and champ at the bit? Nor is he content to vent his spleen on humans alone. Others of the Lord's creatures are objects of his malicious nature, as was shown by an incident which occurred this morning.

At daybreak two small birds came flying over the sea and followed in the ship's wake. They were no bigger in the body than our English robins, but had larger wing spans and longer stem-like legs webbed at the feet. Their upper parts were black and the under parts of a greyish hue. Skimming over the water, they uttered no note or

73

sound and flew so low that at times they would touch the surface and rebound into the air.

Elizabeth called my attention to the birds and we brought some offal and pieces of bread to feed them. It was novel to observe how they partook of the food we cast on the water. A breeze was blowing from the northeast, and the birds would face in the teeth of the wind and flap their wings with a gentle movement to keep the food constantly before them as they ate it. One instant they would be lost to view as they went down in the trough of a wave and on the next they came up with the crest.

We were engaged in this harmless diversion and joined by others of the people who laughed in glee at the birds' antics. Then Shipley was attracted by our merriment, and on seeing the cause he muttered an oath and dashed into the forecastle. In a few moments he emerged with a musket, and before we were aware of his purpose he fired point-blank in the birds' direction. He had taken no aim, yet by chance he found his mark. One of them fell wounded into the sea and the other flew southward with the speed of the wind, chirping as it went.

A cry of dismay welled up from the spectators and I turned on him in anger, demanding: "Why did you do it? The birds were not harming you. Are you so choked with the lust to kill that no living thing can escape you?"

"Those were devil-birds," he answered, scowling across the water. "They're forerunners of ill omen and bring misfortune to a ship's crew. With them in our wake we'd be sure to meet with storms and gales that'd blow the ship to bits and we'd never arrive at haven. We're best rid of them, I tell you."

He spoke with great earnestness, and knowing that seamen the world over are notoriously superstitious I felt inclined to take his sincerity for granted. Then again I thought he had employed this as a pretext to wreak vengeance on the birds as an outlet for the ill will he bears us.

"What have the birds to do with storms and gales?" I scoffed. "It's a foolish notion and no man of the least understanding would pay it any heed."

"Nay, lad," broke in Tom English. "There's a full measure of truth in what he says. Time and again I've seen it borne out. Some four years ago I sailed under Captain Corning in the *Swallow* on a passage to Holland. We had fair weather till two of the devil-birds came flying at our stern. Soon after we were struck by a fearful storm that raged for three days. We were driven from our course and wrecked off the coast of Norway. Two of us were all that were left of the crew to tell the tale. Once before I sailed—"

"Look!" cried someone. "The other bird is coming back."

All eyes glanced across the larboard bow, and on the southern horizon a speck could be discerned moving toward us with astonishing speed. There could be little doubt of it. The bird was returning. Hardly five minutes had elapsed since it had passed from view, yet its flight was so swift that it was soon trailing in our wake again, soaring low over the water as if seeking its lost mate.

Shipley cursed aloud, reloaded his musket, and took careful aim and fired. The minuteness of the bird coupled with its being in motion combined to make it a difficult target. I was elated when he missed. It emitted a cheery "tweet tweet" and danced about unharmed. He continued firing until his store of shot was exhausted, but the bird was not to be driven off.

"A silver ball would bring it down," suggested Tom English.

"There's no silver to spare," growled Shipley. "I have another way to do the trick."

He went to the forecastle and returned with some ratsbane. This he molded in with pieces of bread he tossed in the water for the bird to feed on; but for some reason or other, probably having already eaten its fill, it would not partake of the corrupted food. Shipley raged like a man possessed with madness, shrieking curses on the unoffending creature. The sweat broke out on his forehead and he fairly trembled in a convulsion. Within a short time he was in such a weakened state that Tom English had to help him back to the forecastle.

The bird followed us throughout the day and when darkness began to fall it was still visible, winging its way astern the ship. It is most uncanny. I take little stock in supernatural thoughts, holding them in no more repute than old wives' tales. Yet the bird has flown many miles without tiring and clings to our wake like an avenging fury. Is it an omen of evil as the seamen had said? I still doubt it, yet I must confess my doubt is tinged with belief.

Saturday, September 23, 1620

Early this morning a seaman came to our quarters, inquiring for our physician. I directed him to Dr. Fuller's cabin and lingered to hear his mission.

"Captain Jones sent me to call you," the fellow said. "Tom Shipley is taken down with sickness. He's terrible bad off."

"You have your own ship's physician," replied Dr. Fuller. "Can't Dr. Heale look after him?"

"Aye, but he can't make head nor tail of what ails Shipley. Captain Jones thought you might be willing to lend a hand."

"Tell Captain Jones I've neither the time nor patience to spare for Shipley," grumbled Dr. Fuller, but as the seaman started to leave he called after him: "Wait. I'll not refuse to do an act of Christian charity, even though the man isn't deserving of it. You may say I'll be there presently."

The seaman trudged off, and Dr. Fuller said to me: "Lad, ask Will Butten to accompany me to the forecastle. Shipley is sick. I trust it's the pox that has him in its grip."

The last was uttered with great fervency of spirit and inwardly I added an "amen". Then having delivered his message, I went to see if the bird could be sighted. I was imbued with the feeling that in some way or other it was connected with Shipley's sudden attack of sickness. Try as I would, the thought could not be dislodged. On deck the bird was nowhere to be sighted and I must admit breathing a sigh of relief.

A mass of grey clouds was visible in the sky to the northward and reached from east to west across the horizon in a limitless expanse. It was moving southward rapidly. Flashes of lightning forked into the sea and distant claps of thunder echoed and re-echoed in rumbles of discord. I inferred a storm was brewing and sought confirmation from Tom English who, with others of the seamen, had just partly reefed the sail.

"Nay, not a storm, lad," he replied. "The wind's pace has not quickened, nor are those storm clouds. When the wind whistles past your ear like the snap of a lash and the clouds are thick and black as darkest night, then's the time you'll know a storm is brewing. We're likely to have rain; it's long past due. But there'll be no storm today."

I then asked: "What ails Tom Shipley?"

The seaman shook his head dubiously. "He was taken down with a fever last night and went clean out of his head raving about the devil-birds. This morning he's worse. He can't move body nor limb. Those cursed birds brought it on him, I'll warrant. It's God's own blessing they're both gone or they'd bring us more mischief."

I was more inclined to consider Shipley's illness in the light of a just retribution rather than a mischief, but I held my peace. The clouds were sailing overhead and a moderate rain was falling. It came down with a gentle patter, leaving moist imprints that seeped into the dry wood as rapidly as it touched the deck. The air was refreshing and I inhaled deeply before going below.

In about half an hour Dr. Fuller returned from the forecastle with his brow wreathed in furrows. The news of Shipley's sickness had spread through the Company, and he was beset by a throng of inquisitors who clamored to hear the details. He volunteered no information more than to say that the fellow was in a desperate condition.

"What's the nature of his ailment?" demanded Stephen Hopkins.

"I'll not say," replied Dr. Fuller.

"Do you think he'll recover?" he persisted.

"I'll not answer at present."

"I'll not say and I'll not answer," mocked Stephen Hopkins. "Here's a fine kettle of fish for you. A man is taken sick and the physician will not report what ails the patient, or if he'll live or die. What a comfort to know that the welfare of our people is in such able hands. I'll venture to say you're so close-lipped for the reason that you don't know what the affliction is."

The shrewd guess he had hazarded brought a trace of color to Dr. Fuller. "Have it your way then, Mr. Hopkins," he said as he withdrew into his cabin.

Stephen Hopkins' opinion was confirmed later when I talked to Will Butten. "Do not repeat it, John," he said, "but Shipley is afflicted with a strange malady that is not known either to Dr. Fuller or Dr. Heale. Dr. Fuller thinks it may be the lux or scurvy, yet in some ways it's different. He's at a complete loss for a remedy or how to treat Shipley. Dr. Heale even fears to go near the patient. He's washed his hands of the case and left it in Dr. Fuller's sole charge."

It was startling to hear that a man in the soundest health had been brought so low overnight. Yesterday Shipley was lusty and robust; today he is scorched and blighted. Is it not a manifest example of the uncertainty of our mortal existence? I will not gloat over his misfortune, yet there is good cheer in the thought that for a time we shall have relief from his harassments. Yea, the Lord in His wisdom is infinite and His ways surpass human understanding.

Sunday, September 24, 1620

Truly this was the first peaceful Sabbath Day we had known aboard ship and it was given unto rest and communion with the Lord of Hosts. All were on deck except Isaac Allerton and John Billington. The former stayed in his cabin nursing his wound, and Billington was still under sentence of confinement on bread and water.

Before the services got under way Stephen Hopkins accosted John Carver and solemnly declared: "Mr. Carver, the London people have been sadly troubled. Here we're on the high sea with no pastor of our own to minister to our spiritual needs. This is a sore affliction and we've been feeling it keenly. I've given considerable thought to the matter. After all, what's a mere difference in the form of religion between you of Leyden and us? We all worship the same God and His Son, the Prince of Peace. And so, in behalf of the London people and myself, I humbly petition that we may be granted leave to join with you in prayer services."

I gasped and held my breath, somehow suspecting a hidden motive behind his pious expression.

"Mr. Hopkins, your words are gratifying beyond measure," John Carver warmly responded. "If the action of the London people follows suit, it will help bind us into a more compact unity. Surely no one need petition to raise his voice in prayer to the Almighty. It is for this priceless boon that we accepted exile in Holland and now seek refuge across the sea. Freedom to worship God in accordance with one's conscience is an inalienable right not only of freemen but of felons as well. None should be deprived of it."

"If that's the case then there's no reason why John Billington shouldn't be allowed to join with us," said Stephen Hopkins with the calm assurance of a man who has gained his point. "Should he be deprived of his inalienable right to worship?"

The jack was now out of the box, and I felt some relief in the thought that Stephen Hopkins had justified my suspicion.

"If the man wishes to partake of worship," announced John Carver coldly, "he is welcome to do so."

John Billington was brought up to join us in prayer and sought to make the most of his opportunity. He was tumultuous in his pious incantations, stirring himself into a frenzy of repentance and crying out in abject humility for the Lord's forgiveness. He played his part well and drew favorable comment from many of the London people.

"Mark how Billington conducts himself," Stephen Hopkins whispered to me. "Did you ever before see so penitent a sinner? I'm convinced the spirit of godliness has entered into him. What's your thought in the matter, lad?"

I nodded in assent, though in so doing I belied the truth of my belief. Billington's show of retribution did not impress me overly. I feared it was all a sham. The man is an arrant rogue of the first water, and once he has gained his release he will again stand revealed for the base profligate that he is.

The services were concluded with Elder Brewster's benediction. After giving thanks to the Lord for having brought us thus far on our voyage without casualties, he pleaded for Isaac Allerton's recovery and even for Tom Shipley to be forgiven his iniquities and restored to a sound body. And all the people said, "Amen."

Monday, September 25, 1620

Isaac Allerton's wound mends apace, but it is otherwise with Tom Shipley. He is at a low ebb. I went to the forecastle this morning with Dr. Fuller and Will Butten to see his condition. He was lying on a bed abounding in filth and with nothing but vermin for company. His body is marked with spots of an ash-copper hue. Between his fingers and on parts of his face the skin is parched and cracked open, leaving the naked flesh bared to view. He presented so hideous a spectacle that it was all I could do to restrain myself from fleeing his presence.

He moved his head in our direction and rolled his eyeballs like a caged beast. "Water," he moaned. "Water."

"Quick, Will, some water," cried Dr. Fuller. "I dare say the poor fellow's had nothing to drink all night."

He aided him to a sitting posture while Will hastened for a cup of water. Shipley clutched it in both hands with barely enough strength to raise it to his lips and sip slowly. After finishing he handed it back to Will and reclined with his eyes closed.

"How is my patient faring today?" inquired Dr. Fuller cheerfully as he felt Shipley's pulse.

I marveled at the physician's courage. I would not have touched the spotted limb for all the gold in Cathay.

Shipley shook his head.

"Where are the seamen?" demanded Dr. Fuller. "Can't they at least bring you some water in your distressed condition?"

The seaman's eyes opened and lit up in a blaze of fury. "The rogues deserted me." He spoke with difficulty and interspersed each sentence with vehement curses. "They were my friends when I was well. Now that I lie sick they'd leave me die like a rat in a trap. They'll not raise a finger to help me."

"Never fear," said Dr. Fuller. "I'll see to it that one of us visits you every so often so's you'll want for nothing. We'll do our utmost for you."

Shipley mumbled his thanks and turned his head to the wall. No doubt he was reflecting over our returning good for all the evil he had done us.

"Have you eaten anything since I was here last night?" asked Dr. Fuller.

He again shook his head. Dr. Fuller made him show his tongue, and it appeared black and considerably swollen.

"Will, his passage is so choked that I doubt if he can eat coarse food," said Dr. Fuller. "Go to my cabin and bring back a confection of conserves."

When Will returned with the conserves, Dr. Fuller dissolved it in water and braced Shipley in an upright position to enable him to partake of the sustenance. He swallowed it in small gulps under evident hardship, but did not leave off until the last drop was gone.

"Do you feel somewhat better now?" inquired Dr. Fuller.

This time he responded with an affirmative nod and was asleep in a few minutes. There being nothing more to be done for him, we left. Outside the forecastle a number of seamen, including Robert Coppin, the pilot, approached us and inquired somewhat timidly as to Shipley's condition.

"Go in and see for yourselves," replied Dr. Fuller curtly.

"I'll not set foot in there," responded Robert Coppin. "It's the pestilence he has and I'll not run the risk of being tainted from him."

"Nor I," grumbled one of the seamen, and the others expressed like sentiments.

"You are his friends, yet you show indifference to his welfare," said Dr. Fuller. "You'll not as much as extend yourselves to bring him water when he calls for it. Then what need you expect from us who are no friends of his?"

"You're a physician," answered Robert Coppin. "We have no protection against the sickness, but you can ward it off yourself."

"Misguided man," said Dr. Fuller in a pitying tone. "It's true I'm a physician, yet I can perform no miracles for myself. My profession has its risks and I must look them in the face without flinching. But I can no more prevent myself from getting sick than I can keep the sun from rising or setting."

"How is Shipley getting along?" insisted Robert Coppin.

"Oh, as well as can be expected."

"Will he recover?"

"That I can't answer with certainty."

"He'd best be quick about it one way or the other," growled a seaman. "It's dreadful poor sleeping these chill nights, what with him keeping us away from our warm beds."

"Aye," added another, with an evil glint in his eyes. "It would be a discretion to cast him overboard, pestilence and all, before we're tainted with it. Why need we risk our lives for him? Out of the way with him, I say."

We walked off from them, followed by surly threats which boded ill for Shipley.

"They display the true breeding of wolves," remarked Dr. Fuller. "They'd dispatch a sick comrade before his eyes are closed in death. Fortunately they'll be spared the vile deed. I doubt if Shipley will live more than a day or two at the most. His mortal hours are numbered."

He spoke with a calm assurance that startled me. I have ever entertained a horror of death. The mere suggestion of it alone suffices to freeze the blood in my veins. Now it was extending a long arm over many leagues of sea to pluck a victim from our midst while we must stand by helpless.

Nor was this all. On land a deceased could be laid to rest in firm soil where near ones and dear ones might come to shed a tear over the departed. But here at sea there could be nothing except a watery grave, unmarked and unhallowed. It is awful to contemplate. May the Lord have mercy on Shipley and spare him this dire fate.

Tuesday, September 26, 1620

Isaac Allerton came on deck this forenoon for the first time since he had been wounded. He was somewhat pallid and had his head swathed in a bandage, though otherwise he seemed in a fair state of health. The people greeted his appearance with an outpouring of congratulations. It was a happy moment and all joined in expressing their joy over his recovery.

Stephen Hopkins delivered a pompous address appropriately suited to the occasion and then beckoned to John Carver, saying: "I would have a word with you. No doubt you've observed that Isaac Allerton has recovered from his hurt?"

"I have," answered John Carver, "and I'm well pleased with it."

"And I likewise," said Stephen Hopkins. "But now that he's recovered there's no need to keep John Billington confined on bread and water any longer. The man's atoned for his sin. Did you observe how he demeaned himself at the services this past Sabbath? I'll warrant he'll toe the mark henceforth and be a credit to us."

John Carver frowned. "I'll discuss it with the Elders later in the week."

"And meanwhile Billington lies in durance vile like a beast in a dungeon," cried Stephen Hopkins. "Is this just,

I ask you? Should he be forced to suffer torture while you dally over it with the Elders? Nay, Mr. Carver. I petition you in a gentle way for his release. If that does not suffice, then the London men must seek redress by a harsher method. It irks them sorely that one of their own should be secluded from the light of day for so long a time."

"He's been confined only since last Thursday," protested John Carver. "Hardly five days have gone by."

"Yet five days can be lengthened into as many years when a man is denied his freedom."

"That is true. I'll summon the Elders to meet at once. No doubt your point will be well taken."

"It best had be," said Stephen Hopkins grimly.

"I'll not be coerced by you," cried John Carver. "If Billington is released it will be for the sake of justice and not because of your threats."

"Threats?" Stephen Hopkins' moon-round face assumed a bland expression of surprised innocence. "I uttered no threats. I merely said I thought it would be best to release him. Where is there any threat in that?"

"Very well then, Mr. Hopkins."

As John Carver stalked off, Stephen Hopkins chuckled audibly. "There he goes, the old coxcomb," he remarked to me. "See how he walks past the people with his nose in the air as if they taint the very air he breathes. I've heard it said he's to be chosen our governor. A likely man indeed for the office. Why the people would rise up in rebellion against him in no time."

I protested his sour declarations, and he hastened to say: "Oh, no offense, lad, take no offense. John Carver is a worthy man, a most worthy man for the proper purpose. He'll see to it that Billington is released forthwith. Now you mark what I say."

His words were borne out within the hour when Billington, blinking like an owl, was escorted on deck a freeman. Stephen Hopkins and many of the Londoners gathered about and gave him a welcome like the homecoming of the Prodigal Son. I turned away from the noisy demonstration. It could serve no good purpose and would only encourage the fellow to resume his dissolute ways.

At noonday I went with Dr. Fuller to bring some broth for Shipley. We found him well nigh a corpse, lying on his back and staring vacantly. His jaws were clamped so tightly that Dr. Fuller could hardly pry them apart to force some of the broth down his throat. His body is soot black and his eyes creep from his forehead. A loathsome sight, and he cannot survive.

As we were leaving the forecastle Captain Jones hailed us and inquired about Shipley's condition. When advised thereof by Dr. Fuller, he said he would be sorry to lose him. The fellow is an able-bodied seaman and there might be need for his brawn before the voyage is over. But Dr. Fuller can do nothing more and gave the captain scant hope of Shipley's recovery.

Wednesday, September 27, 1620

Tom Shipley is no longer of this world. He surrendered the ghost an hour before sundown. Will Butten brought the news of his death, and out of curiosity's sake I accompanied Dr. Fuller who went to confirm the report. Captain Jones and his crew were assembled in force outside the forecastle. The seamen were speaking in hushed tones and cringed in awe as we passed them. The captain nodded to Dr. Fuller who returned the salute with a like motion.

We entered the forecastle, followed by the seamen at a cautious distance to our rear. The corpse presented the most gruesome spectacle I had ever beheld. The sightless eyes were wide open and the lips had shrunk back from the yellowish teeth so that for all the world his features resembled a grinning death's-head. The body was so rotted and wasted that I thought it would crumble to the touch. An overpowering odor emanated from it, a foul, offensive stench of decaying animal matter.

"His travail is over," said Dr. Fuller softly.

I stared at the earthly remains of what had once been a man in his prime. It was unbelievable. Less than a week ago he had been a vision of strength and vigor, yet there in his place were so many pounds of flesh and bones soon to be withered to dust. What a transformation! I could not shed any tears over him, but in that awful moment I was overwhelmed by the realization that some day I, too, would be nothing but flesh and bones waiting to be turned into dust.

The sickly thought combined with the rank atmosphere to produce a noxious sensation at the pit of my stomach. The walls of the forecastle seemed to close in on me, black specks floated before my eyes and I felt my legs giving way. Then all was darkness. When I regained consciousness I was thankfully aware that I had been removed from the death chamber and its horror. I was lying on the deck with Dr. Fuller pressing a cup of water to my lips and the seamen standing about in a circle.

"Are you feeling better?" asked Dr. Fuller.

I nodded, and he continued: "I shouldn't have let you stay in there so long. Hardened as I am to sights like that, it was all I could do to keep my own senses, so it's a small wonder you swooned. Let's get you back to your cabin."

One of the seamen helped him to set me upright.

"Shipley is dead then?" inquired Captain Jones. He said it in a matter-of-fact tone, more as a declaration than an interrogation.

"There isn't the least doubt of it," replied Dr. Fuller. "He's breathed his last."

A moment of awkward silence ensued before Captain Jones spoke again. "He was a first-rate seaman, poor fellow, and now he's gone. There's nothing more we can do except give him as decent a burial as we're able, and that'll be a poor one at best. I thank you for what you've done, Dr. Fuller."

"No thanks are needed. I did my utmost and only regret I was unable to save him. But he was beyond all earthly help from the first moment the affliction seized him."

"Aye, so it seemed," the captain muttered. "It was surpassing weird the way he perished. I've never seen the equal in all the years I've sailed the seas."

I stayed in my cabin until Will Butten called me to witness the burial. It was a solemn, awe-inspiring proceeding held at the ship's stern. The rays of the setting sun played on the grave features of our people and the terror-stricken countenances of the seamen. The corpse had been sewed in canvas and weighted with ballast. After a brief prayer by Captain Jones, it was dropped overboard and went down into the sea, fathom after fathom, and the water seethed and churned as the monsters of the deep followed hard after their prey as far as the eye could see.

So has he ended this life. Yea, and so some day we all must be called to meet our Maker. But it please God, in not so desperate a fashion. And Tom Shipley, for all his curses of our people, was himself the first to be cast into the sea.

Thursday, September 28, 1620

I passed a hideous night replete with dreams of Shipley and monstrous sea ogres. His staring eyes penetrated into my sleep and conjured up malignant visions of evil at my bedside. I struggled in their clutches and tried to scream for help, yet even while sleeping I was aware that my shouts seldom rose above a whisper. Several times when it seemed I was being shaken by the furies, it proved to be Will Butten who was arousing me from my distressed slumber to complain that my moans and outcries were keeping him awake.

The last time he awoke me was shortly before daybreak, and rather than suffer further torment I arose and went on deck. The outlook was bleak and dreary in the grey of the morning. The skies were overcast with leaden clouds and the sea was lashed into slate-hued waves topped with white foam. A raw, biting wind was bearing down from the north. Within a few minutes I was chilled to the bone and went below to my cabin.

The weather held miserable, though it later warmed sufficiently to allow us to go on deck. The day was as dull as the weather with nothing to relieve the irksome hours except discourse on subjects of interest. As can readily be imagined, the major discussion centered on Tom Shipley.

The people have forgotten his misdeeds and are filled with pity for him. There was much conjecture as to whether he had left a wife and little ones in England to wait in vain for his return, but none could offer any enlightenment.

His death has wrought a marvel with the seamen. They are amazed over it and believe the wrath of the Lord came upon him for his vile abuse of our people. Where they had been proud and overbearing, they now are most contrite in deadly fear for their own safeties and seek to make amends by every act and show of kindness. Yea, the captain, his mates and the mariners are all humility. They strive to outdo each other in our service, and if their friendship lasts it will ease the burden of our woes for the rest of the voyage.

Friday, September 29, 1620

After another night made wretched by hideous visions of Shipley, I arose and idled the morning away. In the forenoon Captain Jones sent us some dried neats' tongues as a gesture of good will, I take it, and Mrs. Carver cooked them to be served as a relish for our dinners. Before they were apportioned, Captain Jones called with his first mate John Clarke to pay us a visit. An affable discourse ensued. Following this, Stephen Hopkins invited them to partake of the repast.

"Aye, I'll take a bite or so," said Captain Jones.

"If you take more than a bite, then I'd prefer that you'd sew," remarked Stephen Hopkins with a grimace.

The captain and his mate laughed at the quip and ate heartily, so much so that by the time their hungers were appeased there was little of the tongue left for us. Nonetheless we were well pleased with their display of friendship; that is, all except Stephen Hopkins.

When they took their departure he glowered wrathfully after them and grumbled: "There they go, the villainous gluttons. They send us neats' tongues, and after it's cooked to the king's own taste they come on a flimsy pretext and devour it before our eyes. A plague take them and their kind. Couldn't they have delayed their visit till past noonday? And what hungers they brought with them! All I have to say is that if their stomachs go with their friendship, then I'd as soon forfeit both and I'll be the richer by it."

Otherwise the day was uneventful, but the evening was marred by a distressing incident. It was nothing less than strife between Edward Dotey and Edward Leister, both servants to Stephen Hopkins and the dearest of friends since early boyhood. Indeed, aboard ship their tender regard for each other had caused them to be likened to David and Jonathan. Yet what power a vain female holds over the hearts of men to sway friend against friend in brutal combat. And what a scandal to our people. And all because of Mrs. Carver's distant kinswoman, the vixen, Desire Minter.

I did not learn till later how it had started. It seems that on deck past nightfall Edward Dotey found her in the company of Edward Leister. Then each claimed her for his own betrothed and harsh words gave birth to harsher blows. Thus it came about that friend smote friend with might and main, and meanwhile the artful wench pranced about giving vent to pithy shrieks which encouraged them all the more to do each other violence.

The startling news was brought to Stephen Hopkins and he hurried to the scene with a number of us in his trail. No moon was out; it was pitch dark at the ship's stern where the scuffle raged. In the glare of lantern light the friends were discerned at each other's throat in furi-

ous onslaught. They failed to heed Stephen Hopkins'
command to desist and it was much ado for us to wrest
them apart.

"Ned Dotey, Ned Leister," cried Stephen Hopkins in
amazement. "What has come over you that you lust for
each other's blood? What has come between your friendship to have caused this to happen? Answer me."

"He has wronged and injured me," complained Edward Dotey.

"What have you done?" Stephen Hopkins sternly demanded of Edward Leister.

"Nothing," he replied. "He's the one to blame. He has
wronged and injured me, not I him."

Stephen Hopkins glanced from one to the other in
perplexity. "You both say the other has wronged and
injured you. Tell me how."

"I'll say nothing more," remarked Edward Dotey sul-
lenly.

"Nor will I," said Edward Leister.

Stephen Hopkins called the maid Desire Minter.

"You know what caused this. Now speak," he demanded.

"I'm not to blame," she averred with a defiant toss of
the head.

"I did not say you were to blame," he replied. "But it's
evident that they may have good cause for concealing the
truth, and it's known to you. Now what is it?"

She smirked prettily and responded: "I had secretly

plighted my troth to Ned Leister. Then Ned Dotey harried me for my affections and I did not know which of them I preferred. Am I to blame if they came to blows over it?"

Her disclosure was followed by an interval of tense silence. Then Edward Leister, the gentler of the two friends, cried to her: "I'll have nothing more of you. Ned Dotey is welcome to have you if he wishes. But you've left me a gaping wound that will never heal."

Also wroth with her, Edward Dotey said: "Why did you not tell me you had first plighted your troth to Ned Leister? You are faithless like Delilah. I'll not have you for my wife either, and no man will ever woo you."

"Now make your peace with each other," said Stephen Hopkins, "and never allow a fickle wench to come between your friendship."

It was a joyous sight to see the friends embrace in love and affection, and the people applauded with a loud acclaim. As for the maid, she withdrew with great shamefacedness. She had set two weak strings to her bow, yet both snapped in the hour of stress and she would have fared better if she had placed her faith in a single strong one.*

---

* Historical Note: Edward Dotey and Edward Leister fought a duel with cutlasses and knives soon after landing at Plymouth, New England. Desire Minter later returned to England unmarried.

Saturday, September 30, 1620

A black sheep cannot grow white fleece, nor can the profligate John Billington attain virtues alien to his licentious nature. Great evil will come of him, and it is a matter of grave concern to the Elders. From early daybreak till long past nightfall he is daily at the forecastle in fellowship with the seamen. They game and drink together while they truck vile tales and make revelry with ribald songs. In one way it is cause for thanksgiving to be relieved of his odious presence, yet it is a shameful reflection that one of our Company disports himself in so dissolute a manner.

But the sharper woe comes of his bestirring the men of London to disputations with the people of Leyden. He has set up Stephen Hopkins as the proper man to be governor of our new commonwealth, though he well knows that the Leyden people, together with some of the Londoners, have the most voices and favor John Carver for this high office. In this fashion he plays the demagogue and sows seeds of dissension which will bear bitter fruit, and we are likely to reap the harvest any day.

John Carver waited this morning to intercept him in the passageway and asked: "Where are you bound so early?"

"I'm going on deck," replied Billington.

"You're concealing the truth," said John Carver. "You're bound for the forecastle, are you not?"

"What if I am? There's no harm in that."

"No harm in that?" cried John Carver. "You carouse with the seamen and bring disgrace on our heads, and yet you say there's no harm in it? You had best give some thought to the mending of your ways. Let alone the people, you set a most unworthy example for your own two sons. Should they follow in your wayward footsteps, they'll have good cause some day to blame the father who steered them from the beaten path of virtue."

"I'll thank you to leave me rear my children as I see fit," shouted Billington in a rage. "Furthermore my ways are my own and I needn't account to you for them. It's no affair of yours, Mr. Carver."

"It is an affair of mine as it is for all our people," answered John Carver. "Your conduct is of such unbecoming dignity as to cast aspersions on all of us. I warn you that we'll not tolerate it."

"I'm a freeman born and you seek to enslave me and deprive me of my liberties," he cried. "I'll not brook your restraints. I'm a loyal subject to King James of England, God bless him, and I'm not to be fettered by you Leyden Dutchmen. I'll resist you to the utmost, so you'd best have a care how you meddle with me."

Several of the Londoners were attracted by his outcries and drew closer while the dispute was in progress. They applauded Billington's statements. Stephen Hopkins had come out in his nightshirt and he broke in, saying: "Well spoken, John Billington. Well spoken indeed."

"Come now, Mr. Hopkins," said John Carver in a chiding tone. "You're a man of substance. Surely you don't put your stamp of approval on his misconduct."

"Misconduct is it?" replied Stephen Hopkins. "You may call it that if you wish, but I say it's all in the point of view. Here's John Billington going about his affairs and disturbing no one. If he prizes the companionship of seamen above yours or mine, where do we have cause to complain? And what if he does game and drink with them. I say it's his privilege and neither you nor anyone else has the right to dictate to him to the contrary."

"I don't dictate to him," answered John Carver, considerably nettled. "I merely ask that he refrain from setting an evil example for the people."

"Evil to those who evil think," retorted Stephen Hopkins. "You Leyden people have set a rigid standard, and if one should digress a hair from it you cry out, 'It is sinful, it is evil.' If the truth must be told you sin more than you're sinned against. With your pious hypocrisies you've coerced yourselves into a mode of life resting on a sandy foundation. Human emotions and desires cannot be pent in without seeking an outlet, and if that is sealed then beware the deluge when the flood bursts. Nay, Mr. Carver. You may guide yourselves by your ordained precepts, but do not try to compel others to abide by them."

"We seek to compel obedience only to that which

affects the common welfare," said John Carver. "People the world over are governed by laws and regulations which concern the interests of all, not the few. Each individual who is part of a commonwealth owes a duty to his fellowmen to comport himself so as to be above reproach. Else, if every man were given a free rein we would have no government or civil rule."

"That may be, Mr. Carver, but here we are on the high seas bound for a land where there is no law or order and we must establish our own. What is to guide us in this? Are we to be ruled by the unnatural concepts of your Leyden people or by the more human requisites of the Londoners? Answer me that."

"We're to be ruled by what the major part deems just and equitable."

"Granted. Yet the lesser part should not be oppressed with an iron hand and have its liberties stifled. Besides, have we as a body been availed the opportunity to express our sentiments? It may be for all I know that the major part of our people is not in accord with your stringent policies. When we've all had a voice in choosing our governor, then we'll know what's in the minds of the people, and not before then."

"You've not been chosen governor yet, Mr. Carver," interposed John Billington. "Nor will you be, if the London people have their say about it. Stephen Hopkins, now he's a likely man for our governor. What do you say to it, men?"

His appeal evoked a hearty response from the London-ers and an ingratiating smile from Stephen Hopkins.

"Are we to allow the Leyden people to trample us underfoot?" continued Billington.

A chorus of "Nay!" resounded in answer.

"You see how the wind blows, Mr. Carver?" remarked Stephen Hopkins.

"Only too well," he mournfully responded. "I rue the day when your London people joined with us on this voyage. We'd have fared better as one compact body without your disgruntled faction."

He walked off amidst a volley of jeers and taunts. It was to Stephen Hopkins' credit that he rebuked his fol-lowers for their ill-chosen words, saying: "We'll have none of that, men. Let's give the devil his due. John Carver is an upright man and I for one admire him for his qualities, though I don't approve his principles. For his years alone he merits your reverence in place of your jeers."

"He'd best leave us in peace then," growled Billington. "But never fear, Mr. Hopkins. You'll be chosen gov-ernor, and not him. The Londoners are with you to the last man and some of the Leyden people are not averse to you. I've had a nip with them now and then and I've sounded them out. We'll carry it off for you when the time comes."

His words rang like the death knell of our hopes and struck terror in me. Stephen Hopkins as our chief officer would not of itself be the direst misfortune that could befall us, for despite his failings he is sound and, as John Carver had stated, a man of substance. What I fear most, if he should be chosen governor, is that he will heed the counsel of John Billington and other Londoners of a like ilk, and it will beyond doubt bring us to the brink of ruin.

On second reflection there seemed little likelihood that it would ever come to pass. Not all of the London people are in support of Stephen Hopkins; some are in wholesome accord with us. As for Billington's claim that some of the Leyden people favor Stephen Hopkins, I strongly doubt its truth. It may be they cozened him with fair words into this belief, yet it cannot possibly bear the weight of their convictions. But we shall see in the due course of time.

Sunday, October 1, 1620

The new month was ushered in by a calm and peaceful Sabbath Day. It is most impressive and awesome at sea on the Sabbath, and man fears to stand before the Lord except in his true light. League upon league without surcease the ocean frets and foams and churns into froth, forsooth a vast and infinite expanse which is a great miracle and a show of His handicraft.

The heaven is tinted with a royal blue and extends on and on to the distant horizon to mate with the sea. It reposes in majestic solitude, exalted and hallowed, a fit abode for the Supreme Ruler and whence He may gaze down on our craft and hearken to our prayers and psalms to His greater glory.

Confronted by these manifestations of His omnipotent hand, mankind cannot help but be brought to a humble and lowly contemplation of its mean station. Yea, what is man but a grain of sand on the shore, a drop of rain in the sea, a mite of dust in the air? And yet he is created in the image of the Lord and exceedingly precious in His eyes.

Shortly past sundown the wind veered sharply and black clouds assembled to the northward in an ominous array. Nearer and nearer they drifted, giving vent to occasional claps of thunder reverberating over the sea like mighty outbursts of anger from the skies. Darkness descended rapidly and engulfed the twilight. In a short time it was impossible to distinguish objects beyond a stone's throw, and the fairness of the day was blotted out completely.

"All hands aloft to reef the sail," bawled Captain Jones.

The seamen flew up, clinging like spiders to the masts and spars as they feverishly labored with deft hands to furl the sail. It snapped and crackled in their grasp as if in opposition to being confined in traces. The darkness thickened every instant. Seamen and sail were soon lost to view and the pitch black darkness of night swooped down on us.

"A storm is brewing," shouted Captain Jones to us. "All of you below deck."

His words carried above the roar of the wind, though the warning was hardly needed. Most of the people had scurried to their cabins for shelter at the first sign of foul weather. Along with a few of the bolder lights I had stayed above to witness at close range the display of wrath by the elements, but we now abandoned this foolhardy design and went below to await the approaching tempest.

Monday, October 2, 1620

Late last night the storm broke. Nature unleashed her pent-up forces in one gigantic outburst, and we huddled in our cabins white-eyed in terror as the furies shrieked and raged about us. Cross winds blew from every point of the compass with a violence that rattled our cabins and threatened to rend asunder the walls standing as a safeguard between us and the turbulent sea. Rain beat down in torrents. The ship was swept by heavy waves which poured down the hatchway and flooded our cabins. And the thunder rumbled steadily like the rat-tat-tat of a monstrous war drum.

The din and uproar of the storm were enhanced by the piercing cries of women and the wailing of frightened children. It was distracting to hear their voices raised in anguish, yet nothing could be done to allay their fears. The water rose in our cabins till we floundered ankle deep and it still seeped in with no sign of lessening. Then some of the people became panic-stricken; they opened their cabin doors and shouted: "All is lost. The ship is sinking!"

Others raised their voices high in prayer and cried: "The Lord alone can save us."

It was a night of horrors such as exceeds the power of description. Time and again as the ship keeled on end we believed she was sinking and we would be trapped in our cabins. Several times some of us strove to win our way to the upper deck in hope of getting succor from the seamen, but our efforts were in vain. The deluge of water poured down the hatchway with the power of a dam burst loose and beat us back like straws. On the last sortie a welcome sight greeted our eyes. It was Captain Jones coming toward us and spouting water like a whale.

"Back to your cabins, every mother's son of you," he roared. "There's no danger of sinking, the ship'll weather the storm. But I'll not vouch for your safeties unless you stay in your cabins. Back with you, I say."

He disappeared as he had come, shearing his way through the rampant water like a deity from the depths of the sea. His momentary presence and reassuring words heartened us considerably. We returned to our cabins bearing a measure of composure in our bosoms and awaited the break of day with as much forbearance as we could muster.

When dawn came the storm was raging without abatement; nor did it moderate a whit the whole day long. The waves tossed the *Mayflower* hither and yon at random. Her masts were bathed in sea water, and she heaved and snorted in her throes as she rose and fell like the bobbin on a shuttle. Forsooth, we were forsaken to the wind and the sea, and at the haphazard mercy of the elements.

Tuesday, October 3, 1620

The storm rode high during the past night and into the forenoon today. Near midday there was no prospect of mitigation in the offing, and at this inauspicious time Mrs. Hopkins was brought to bed in travail. With the ship careening like a balky steed, her condition was one of exceeding gravity. The people pressed about Stephen Hopkins' cabin with their features drawn in apprehension for his wife's security and that of the new life soon to arrive. Heads were bowed, eyes were closed in prayer to the Almighty.

And lo! It pleased the Lord that the storm abated somewhat, and while the ship lay in a measure becalmed, the child was born in safety. It gave vent to a lusty wail that rose shrill and piping like a clarion call. Cries of "Hear! Hear!" resounded from the people. The door of the cabin was opened and Dr. Fuller, wreathed in smiles, appeared to announce: "It's a boy, and as strapping an infant as I've ever delivered. Mrs. Hopkins has passed the ordeal in an admirable manner. The child is well and its mother is happy."

The people broke into a tumult of fervent thanksgiving and marveled mightily at this display of His divine providence. Elder Brewster said: "The Lord stayed the storm to comfort the mother and ease the infant soul into the world. So He parted the waters of the Red Sea that the Israelites might pass, and so He stayed the sun from setting at Joshua's entreaty. Let us give thanks to the Lord for His manifold blessings. His mercy endureth forever."

It was a festive occasion. Stephen Hopkins strutted about like a gamecock with wings aflap, and the people gathered around to wish him and his good wife joy and long life for their offspring. Withal the event was not free from sorrow. Many an eye was wet with tears and some of the womenfolk wept aloud as they reflected on the hardship this young life must endure in a strange land before he came to man's estate.

Stephen Hopkins frowned at their woebegone countenances, demanding: "Why do you weep? This is no time for lamentations. Thank the Lord, my wife and child are well and there's far more cause to be merry. Come, we'll drink a toast to the health of my newborn. Ha, Ned Dotey, Ned Leister, where are you hiding, you rascals?"

They wormed their way through the press of the throng to his side.

"Bring out the spirits for our guests," he ordered. "Let all drink to their hearts' content. Mind now, see that you don't stint with it. I'll not have it said I play the miser when my wife presents me with a son."

They bustled about and served the drink with a lavish hand. Cups were raised aloft and all waited for the toast from Stephen Hopkins.

"Here's to my newborn," he declared. "He's not my firstborn, nor is he likely to be my last born, but of all my past born and those yet to be born he alone was intended to be storm born. Yet as the Lord stayed the storm for his coming, so may He stay misfortune from his life through all the years to come."

Preceded by hearty cries of "amen," the drafts were quaffed.

"We'll drink another toast," said Stephen Hopkins. "Fill up the cups again."

"Hold," called John Billington. "You haven't named the infant yet. Let's decide on a name before we drink again."

Many names were proffered for the youngling, but none seemed to meet with approval. Finally Billington said: "I have it. The child was born on the ocean and its name perforce should be Oceanus."

Among others John Carver sniffed in high dudgeon. "Oceanus? What manner of a name is that? There's neither rhyme nor reason for it; it's neither English nor Dutch but heathenish. Go to, John Billington. Surely you must be jesting."

"I'm not jesting," he angrily responded, being inflamed with drink. "I maintain the name is a fit and proper one. Heathenish, say you? Whatever comes from your Leyden Church is Christian and all else you call heathenish. I'll ask Mr. Hopkins to judge if the name is suitable. He's the one to decide, and I'll warrant he'll find it to his liking."

Thus appealed to, Stephen Hopkins meditated briefly, and to curry favor with his man Billington, as I thought, he announced: "I see nothing wrong with the name, Oceanus. On the contrary I deem it a most appropriate one. The child was born on the ocean, and as John Billington says, the name must be Oceanus. So be it."

The name was not to the liking of Mrs. Hopkins. "Nay, Stephen," she said. "Oceanus is not a proper name for our son. Let him be called David so he may find favor in the eyes of the Lord."

"Nay, Bess," he replied, frowning. "Do not cross me in this, for my heart is set on it. Let him be named Oceanus."

She pleaded and lamented, but it was useless. He remained as adamant as unyielding flint and the child was named Oceanus.

The second toast went off lamely. Billington had sped another shaft tipped with venom and injected ill will in place of the friendly feeling. The people disbanded to their cabins and shortly thereafter the storm returned full tilt.

Wednesday, October 4, 1620

The storm rages unabated. For three days now our cockleshell little craft has been exposed to the merciless assault of the elements, and she has been shaken by fierce winds which have loosened her joists and made her leaky. The water seeps in as if she were a sieve. Night and day the mariners' backs are bent to the pumps. The seas run mountain high, sweeping the deck with lusty buffets that make the ship quiver from stem to stern. It is little short of a miracle that she keeps afloat.

Below deck we are in desperate straits. Our cabins are constantly flooded with sea water. It dampens the fires under our pots and we must partake of cold victuals, mainly salted meat, dried fish, Holland cheese and beer or water, where warm sustenance would be far more appealing to the stomach. All our chickens, succumbing singly and in groups, have perished, leaving us without fresh meat aboard ship. Forsooth these are dull, cheerless days, and they give promise of untold miseries which we are likely to have as bedfellows for many a day to come.

To augment our woes John Billington is again kindling sparks of discord. He has noised it about that the Leyden people slighted Stephen Hopkins at the birth of the infant, Oceanus; even more, he has set adrift a rumor that they have put the evil eye on the child. The Londoners absorb his devious whisperings as gospel truth instead of malicious slander, and they are surly and on edge to avenge the alleged wrong to their leader.

As soon as John Carver gained ear of what was in the wind, he lost no time in calling Billington to task. "Graceless wretch," he lashed at him. "How dare you spread false reports that we wish evil to befall an innocent child. Only a depraved mind like yours could breed such thoughts so revolting to all human instinct. Whatever evil you say we wished on the child, may it fall on your head instead."

Billington squirmed as he replied: "I did not say you wished evil on the child. I only repeated what I heard from others. It was some of your own Leyden people, if I'm not mistaken."

"You lie," said John Carver. "There are none so debased, either among the Leyden or the London people. You alone are at the root of it. The harm is beyond mending, but I must warn you to cease all such further talk."

"And who are you to give me orders?" demanded Billington. "You'll not seal my lips. Shall I ask leave of you whether I'm to speak or hold my peace?"

"I did not say you were not to speak. I demand that you stop spreading infamous falsehoods."

"I spread no falsehoods," cried Billington. "Whatever is said or done that fails to meet with your approval is charged against me. I'm the scapegoat for all. Mind now, you'd best cease persecuting me. I'll not put up with your abuse any longer, and neither will Mr. Hopkins nor any of the London people. You've aroused our gorge to the choking point with your insults. We'll rise up in arms against you if need be. And I make no idle boast about it either."

John Carver recoiled from the fellow's threatening air. "There's no need for belligerency. It may be you've been unjustly accused that you defend yourself so sturdily. We'll endeavor to show you more leniency hereafter."

He had spoken in a softened tone, and as he turned his back Billington leered after him in a knowing way, only too well aware that he had dug in with the rowels and drawn blood.

So there we are. The tempest turmoils without and dissension is aflame within, while we are ground between the upper and nether millstones. If we escape one the other threatens us with extinction. Whither are we drifting on this voyage? And to what bitter end? I dare not look too far ahead. Our present store of grief is far too pressing.

Thursday, October 5, 1620

There was a lull in the storm during the past night and we went to bed nursing the fond hope that fair weather would greet us on the morrow. When dawn came the wind had died off and the water was fairly calm, but the weather was extremely dismal. A mist rose out of the sea and enwrapped us in its dense folds. The darkness was so thick it made the day seem like night, and we lit the lamps and lanterns or else we could not see an ell's pace from the nose.

We moped about and waited for the light of day to pierce the haze. Hours dragged by on leaden feet without a rift in the fog; if anything it deepened to an even more fearful pitch of darkness. The unnatural absence of light caused a tremor of apprehension to sweep through the people, and there was a great deal of talk concerning supernatural things and matters beyond the insight of mortals. Some said we had entered a pale of darkness; others thought we had touched the channel flowing to the land bordering on Purgatory.

The grisly discourse put us all more or less in a perturbed frame of mind. The seamen, as can well be imagined, were even more strongly affected by the eerie surroundings. We neither saw nor heard them until some time past midday when they came hurtling pellmell down the hatchway, stampeding in a body and shouting: "The world is ended, the world is ended!"

We were nearly startled out of our wits and for the moment a near panic ensued. Shrieks and outcries rent the air and many of our lesser people were tainted with the seamen's fears and prayed aloud for the salvation of their souls. But as nothing developed, the frenzy gradually subsided and gave way to calmer judgment. The seamen, however, were not to be soothed. They moaned and wailed that this was their last day on earth and the morrow would see them all in another world.

Friday, October 6, 1620

Notwithstanding the seamen's belief to the contrary, we awoke this morning to find ourselves still moored to earth, or rather the sea. It was most disheartening, though, to discover that the mist and fog had not lifted. We seemed to be in a sea of eternal night, and the darkness enshrouded us in a pall of gloom. The *Mayflower* was like a ghost-ship on the brink of eternity, weighted with living souls and perished corpses.

The seamen were prostrated and awaited the clap of doom every instant. We ourselves were none too stanch in spirit either. Depressed and frayed to the core by the ghastly darkness, we sat mewed up in our cabins and trembled at the grotesque images cast by the flicker of burning wicks. These became magnified in the mind's eye and assumed monstrous shapes and forms all out of proportion to the norm. Every least sound swelled in volume and drummed in our ears with animated resonance.

Near midday we were terrified by an outburst of desperate shrieks in the passageway. It issued from Stephen Hopkins' cabin, and we rushed in to learn the cause. There we found Mrs. Hopkins moaning and weeping bitterly in the throes of anguish while her distracted husband pleaded with her to tell what had happened.

Finally she succumbed to his entreaties and said: "I fell asleep with my babe at my breast, and while I slept an evil vision came to me. Two witches rode on a broom from England and flew over the sea into my cabin. One of them took the child from my arms to fondle it and said, 'Sister, what is written in the book of fate for this infant?'

"The other crone answered, 'On the ocean he first saw the light of day. He is named for and bonded to the ocean. If he stays on the ocean, then shall his ventures prosper and he will be a lord of high degree. But if he sets foot ashore, even for a short time, then is he foredoomed to an early grave.' After that they cackled hideously and whisked away."

Stephen Hopkins broke into laughter. "Tut, tut, it's an idle vision and of no repute. Who would take stock in such a fable? No one, I'll warrant, except a foolish woman. Let it pass from your mind, Bess. It's nothing."

But she was like Rachael crying in the wilderness and not to be comforted. "Nay, Stephen, it was my second sight that came to me in the vision. It was an evil day when you named our son Oceanus. I pleaded with you and beseeched you not to do it, but you would not be moved. Why didn't you heed me?"

"The devil take all the witches and keep them for his own," he cried. "Am I to be tormented for the reason that two of them came in a dream and foretold evil for our son? Who ever heard the like of it before? Now be quiet and cease your idle prattling before people will think you're in your dotage."

Elder Brewster spoke more gently to her. "Mrs. Hopkins, visions that come while we sleep are only the workings of a feverish mind. Your mother instinct urges you to dread that misfortune may lie in wait for your newborn in the time to come. But there is nothing to fear, I assure you. Your son's fate is in the hands of the Lord even as with all mankind, and He will deal gently with him. He who does not suffer a sparrow to fall unseen will surely shield him from harm."

"You hear that, Bess," exclaimed Stephen Hopkins. "Now have done with your dream of old crones. I dare say our son will grow to sturdy manhood and be a blessing to us in our old age."

She made a brave attempt to stifle her tears, but as we left the cabin her low sobbing broke out anew. I pitied her and condemned John Billington for the evil he had wrought. Nor did I consider Stephen Hopkins blameless, for he should have been ruled by his wife in naming the child. But after all a name is nothing more than a name and it would be foolish to give weight to ill-omened dreams.*

---

* Historical Note: Oceanus died in infancy at Plymouth, New England, after having been taken off the *Mayflower*.

Saturday, October 7, 1620

Last night a slight breeze came into play and impelled the vapors to swirl in easy motion. Our lights shone free from haze for the first time in two days. By daybreak the fog was completely gone and we rushed on deck to give praise to the Lord for having delivered us from the Egyptian darkness. No body of mortals ever welcomed the light of day with such thanksgiving and heartfelt acclaim.

Our joy, however, was short-lived. The wind quickened its speed and in a short time was blowing a gale of the utmost fury and violence. Coming from the north in fitful gusts, it racked the ship with such fearful blows that we thought she would be rent asunder. The seas were surpassingly high. Monstrous wave after wave swooped down on the *Mayflower* to rake her deck, and her uppers were loosened and made leaky.

The rigging was torn to shreds and the masts, constructed as they were of sturdy green timber, swayed and whipped through the air like reeds in the wind. The mainbeams in the midship were of more ancient wood than the masts and lacked their supple grace. Under the strain of being buffeted by the wind and waves, one of the mainbeams gave indications of splintering early in the day. It finally cracked and gave way in the lower deck, though by the grace of God no one was hurt.

Captain Jones came below with the ship's carpenter to survey the break in the mainbeam. "What's your thought on it?" he asked the carpenter. "Can the damage be repaired?"

"I'll not venture to speak with certainty," he answered. "It could be done with tools and timber, but not without them."

"You have the tools," said the captain hopefully.

"Aye, but where shall I get timber to shape a new mainbeam?"

Captain Jones gave John Carver a troubled glance. "You've heard what the carpenter said," he remarked. "If the beam can't be mended, we'll be in a sorry plight."

"How grave is it then?" asked John Carver.

"It would be a mortal danger for us to go further."

John Carver was appalled at this declaration, and indeed we were all struck speechless with dismay.

"Then the beam must be mended one way or another," he said firmly.

"Aye, but how?" demanded Captain Jones. "If you'll offer a remedy, I'll gladly apply it to best advantage."

"I don't know of any," John Carver admitted. "But the Lord will not desert us in our hour of need. I'm certain He will come to our rescue."

"Then He'd best be quick about it," responded the captain with brash irreverence. "Your faith in Providence is highly commendable, Mr. Carver, but it will take more than faith to replace the broken beam. We can do nothing till the storm blows over, and perhaps by that time a plan will come to light. Otherwise we may be forced back to port."

The shadow cast by this latest casualty steeped us in utter despondency. For a month and a day we had sailed onward in the face of manifold obstacles. We had contended with sickness, abuse from the seamen, wrangles with the London people and the fury of the elements, yet we had not deviated from our course. Now the broken mainbeam stares us in the face and threatens to bring our voyage to naught. But the Lord's will be done. And meanwhile the storm roars on unabated.

Sunday, October 8, 1620

The tempest raged unrelentingly and gave no promise of subsiding. Due to the adverse weather conditions we were forced to dispense with Sabbath Day services in a body, and in lieu thereof the Elders ordained it to be a fast day. Elder Brewster went from cabin to cabin and exhorted us to devote ourselves to prayer and fasting. Most of the people complied, but some of the Londoners grumbled and made a mockery of it.

"Prayer is well enough," said Stephen Hopkins, voicing the opinion of the malcontents. "But what need is there for a special fast day when every day is nothing else? For a week I've been nibbling on dampened cheese like a mouse trapped in a bin. My stomach hungers for warm meat, yet I must eat cheese or starve. I'll fast this day, Mr. Brewster, if you'll promise fair weather and a feast for the morrow."

"How can I promise you that? You know well it's beyond my control."

"Then neither can I promise to fast," averred Stephen Hopkins, "for the very good reason that my stomach is beyond my control. Nay, I'll dine on cheese this day even though it's loathsome to me. Let those fast who are too proud to partake of this humble fare."

Despite this attempted levity, the atmosphere was doleful without a ray of cheer to bolster our depressed spirits. Our chief men were wrestling with the problem of the broken mainbeam. No solution came to mind, though suggestions were proffered thick and fast and each in turn discarded. Yet we have not lost faith in the Almighty, and faith can work miracles when all else has failed.

Monday, October 9, 1620

The miseries brought on by the elements are rapidly surpassing the bounds of our endurance. The storm abated somewhat in the forenoon and we hoped fair weather would ensue. On the contrary, hail as large as hens' eggs clattered down on the deck at midday and following came a deluge of rain that turned to sleet. It was bitterly cold and we dressed warmly, many even wrapping blankets about themselves. Yet without fires to warm our numbed limbs, there was scant comfort for us.

Shivering and snuffling in our damp cabins, we fell prey to the direst apprehensions. We were now in our fifth week of beating at sea and our haven seemed beyond any possible hope of attainment. The unseasonable cold weather called attention to the rapid approach of winter with all its dreaded cohorts. Nothing but snow and frost would await us on our arrival if we ever did outlive the storms and complete the voyage. Nor were we any closer to a solution for the vexatious problem of the broken beam.

Truly there was more than ample cause for the ebbed state of our hopes and anticipations. This was even aggravated past midday when the storm swelled to a pitch of hitherto unattained ferocity and rode rampant for several hours. It was the last upheaval of the spent and exhausted force of nature. By nightfall the storm had blown over and the skies were clear for the first time since a week past Sunday. A measure of relief is in sight for us. We will assuredly have fair weather on the morrow.

Tuesday, October 10, 1620

The day broke clear and fair with the sun coming out ablaze in glory, the first we had seen in eight days. The people poured out on deck to bask in its life-giving rays. A balmy breeze swept in from the southwest and we drank deeply of its fragrant warmth. As it diffused through our veins, the chill fled from our bones to be replaced by a glow of invigoration. Health and life seeped into the gaunt, pallid features of men, women and children, and we gave praise to the Lord for His gifts and blessings.

The seamen were ruefully surveying the wreckage of the ship's rigging and spars. These appeared in a dubious state of disrepair, but as was evidenced by their conversation, they were more gravely concerned with the leaky upper works and the cracked mainbeam.

"We cannot mend it here asea," declared Robert Coppin. "It would be a discretion to tack about and make sail for England. The ship is so weakened she may sink before long."

"Aye," said another. "It would be to our deadly peril to venture further. What need have we to stake our lives for our wages? That'll be of small worth to us if we're dead men. Let's bear up, say I, and sail for England."

The seamen were all of a like tenor, and it troubled us

to hear their expressions without regard for our desires. When Captain Jones appeared, our chief men met to consult with him and his mates as to which course was to be pursued. There was much diversity of opinion and great perplexities arose.

"The seamen are muttering we had best turn back," said John Carver. "What is to hinder us from sailing onward? We've come thus far and survived the storms in safety. Let us have faith in the Lord and proceed on the voyage. What do you say, Captain Jones?"

"It would be a great hazard," he answered, wagging his head. "If the ship should sink and we all go down in her, it would be a bitter cost to pay for our rashness. It may be wiser to turn back while we're still afloat. For all I know we might never reach England, but every league eastward would bring us closer to succor."

"You have lost heart," remarked John Carver. "We thought you to be cast from a sterner mold than to turn tail and flee when our goal is almost in sight. Reconsider your intent, Captain Jones, and let us sail on."

"Nay, you misjudge me," he protested with great vehemence. "For myself, I stand ready to sail on till no part of the ship is above water except the top-most spar. But what of the lives in my charge? If you place no value on the lives of your people, it will be on your heads. But for my own men, I'll have no hand in sending them to face certain death. Nor can you rightfully ask it of them. Their agreement does not call for it."

"It is true," admitted John Carver. "Is the danger so imminent? Is it not possible to avoid this peril if we proceed onward?"

"That I would not answer with certainty," responded the captain. "We could caulk the upper works and I know the ship would be secure in the water. But how are we to mend the mainbeam? I have no wish to return. We're nearly half the sea over by now and the danger lies behind as well as before us. It might be better to go onward."

As Captain Jones wavered, Robert Coppin interposed: "Nay, captain, the storms have made the ship unseaworthy, and if we caulk the uppers it would but stem the tide for a day. With the workings of the ship, she would not keep stanch overly long. And what of the broken mainbeam? It must be replaced, for the upper deck has lost one of its main props, and at the first stress it will give way and the ship be rent in twain."

"Aye, but that's as likely to happen if we bear up for England as well as if we continue to Virginia. Once we arrive there we can get new timber for a mainbeam."

"Yet if the *Mayflower* should give way while we're bound for England we may hail some passing ship to aid us in our distress, while the other way there's no hope of meeting any sail."

The mates held with Robert Coppin, and Captain Jones reluctantly said: "There's no doubt of it. The sounder course would be to face about. Do you agree, Mr. Carver?"

"I hardly know what to say," he answered, his brow clouded in gloom. "Our hearts and fortunes are bound up in this venture. To turn back to port would leave us void of hope and baffled in our sore trials and endeavors. Yet I do not see how we can obstinately hold to our course in the face of firm opinions of our destruction. Many precious lives are intrusted to our care and we cannot suffer them to be exposed to loss. Grant us a few moments to discuss it, if you will."

The Elders went into a harrowing consultation. It was interrupted by Moses Fletcher, a smith from Leyden.

"Mr. Carver," he said, "if caulking the upper works will make the ship safe in sailing, then a solution for the broken mainbeam has come to my mind. I have a large iron jackscrew tucked away in the ship's hold. I'm sure it can wedge the broken mainbeam back into place. We could then fasten the beam with an iron hoop and I'll warrant it will be nearly as sturdy as before."

John Carver hastened to Captain Jones with the plan, and the ship's carpenter was asked what he thought of it.

"It well might be," he replied. "If the jackscrew can force the mainbeam back into place, we can set a smaller beam under it and make it secure. If this is done, we'd be in small jeopardy and can sail on our way with easy minds."

To our unbounded joy Captain Jones also agreed, and we went to work with a will. By midday the task was completed and we resolved to proceed on our voyage, though not wholly without doubts and misgivings. Yet if it had not been for Moses Fletcher and his jackscrew, we might have been forced to turn back and our voyage come to naught.

Wednesday, October 11, 1620

This morning the skies were overcast with black clouds to presage the advent of a fresh storm. After one day of fair weather, we were again to be assailed by the elements. A feeling of despair gripped me and with it was mingled an intense hatred for the sea and all the afflictions it had brought us. Were we never to be afforded relief? I felt inclined to shake my fist in the face of our tormentor.

"Another storm is approaching," I remarked to Will Butten.

He nodded in gloomy assent, and I took note of how peaked and wasted he appeared with his hollow cheeks and dull eyes.

"You're not looking well," I said. "Is anything the matter?"

"Nothing," he answered with a wan smile. "This extended confinement is sapping my strength. You, yourself, are not as robust as you were, and for that matter all the people suffer from the foul weather."

"It can't endure forever," I muttered. "These storms must cease some time. It may be that this one is the last we'll have."

"At least it will serve one good purpose," he said. "It

will test the caulked upper works and the mended main-beam. If they fail to withstand the stress, then it might be prudent to turn back before we've gone too far."

The storm unloosened a heavy downpour of wind and rain. The upper works were made leaky afresh and the water came through in abundance to flood the ship's hold. She listed heavily and threatened to founder, but was kept afloat by the dint of constant pumping. It was somewhat of a comfort, though, that the mended main-beam held firm, yet we were forced to drift with our sail reefed and could make no furtherance.

The foul weather had brought an attack of colds to all the people and in addition discontentment to some of the Londoners. These latter were surly and short-tempered to a marked degree. They fairly spoiled for pretexts to vent their disfavor on all comers and enlivened the day's apathy by numerous wrangles and exchanges of fisticuffs. These were confined to themselves. The Leyden people were too spiritless to engage in quarrels with them, either verbal or otherwise.

Past midday I was summoned to John Carver's cabin and found him with Captain Jones.

"Captain Jones has asked that some of our people be sent to relieve the seamen at the pumps," said John Carver.

"Aye, my men are so worn out they stand ready to fall from exhaustion," added the captain.

"I've chosen a half dozen of our sturdier men to take

their shift at the work," John Carver continued. "Will you bear your share of it?"

I readily assented, and he smiled in his gracious way, saying: "Very well then. And will you ask Stephen Hopkins to spare me a few moments?"

I was tempted to state that Stephen Hopkins would doubtless take no part in so irksome a task, but it did not seem likely that John Carver wished him for this purpose, and I went to do his bidding.

"He wants me at his cabin, does he?" responded Stephen Hopkins with a sour expression. "Why doesn't he come here if he wishes to see me? I'm not at his beck and call. What ails the worthy Mr. Carver?"

"Captain Jones has called for men to relieve the seamen at the pumps—"

"What!" he interposed, springing up flushed with anger. "Is that what he wants me for—for pumping? The beggarly old he-goat. I'll pump him full with all the woe and misery stored within me. I'll stuff his insulting words down his throat till he chokes on them. I'll—"

"Hold, Mr. Hopkins," I cried as he ranted on. "I did not finish yet. I was about to say that I did not think he wanted you for that."

"Then what else?" he demanded.

"I don't know."

"It hardly matters. Whatever it may be, it holds no interest for me. I'll not go to see him. If he wishes to see me, I dare say he can find his way to my cabin."

I took the message to John Carver. His eyebrows arched higher in a slightly inquiring expression.

"Then I shall go to see him," he said.

As he entered, Stephen Hopkins fell to berating him. "How now, Mr. Carver. Since when am I your menial that you order me to do your pumping? Are there no bounds to the indignities you heap on my head? I'll not lift a finger to pump a stroke though the ship sinks. Now that's an end to it."

John Carver stared dumfounded at him. "John," he said to me, "did you tell Mr. Hopkins that I wanted him to work at the pumps?"

"Oh, he's not to blame," Stephen Hopkins quickly interposed. "He said nothing, but I inferred it. What else would you need me for, except something distasteful?"

"You are far too hasty in your judgment," declared John Carver. "Captain Jones has asked us to relieve his men at the pumps. I've assigned six of the Leyden men to this duty and it's no more than proper that some of the Londoners should also take a hand in it."

"I'll not ask any of them," he snapped. "We've eaten nothing but the bread of affliction since we left Plymouth. We've been abused and downtrodden by you and yours. When matters of importance are in the wind, my counsel is neither asked nor heeded, but when it comes to drudgery, then you wish me to employ my good offices in your behalf. Let the Leyden people pump away for dear life till they're blue in the face. It's no concern of mine."

"When have we refused to heed your counsel?" asked John Carver.

"When have you asked for it, let alone heeded it?" stormed Stephen Hopkins. "Only yesterday you put your heads together and almost decided we should sail back to England. Did you come and say, 'Stephen Hopkins, what is your opinion?' You did not. I sold my properties in London and staked a good round sum in this venture, far more than most of your beggarly Leyden people. If we turned back I stood to lose all by it. Yet you play fast and loose with what concerns the purse of another without so much as consulting him."

"It might have been a discretion to return, the way it stood yesterday."

Stephen Hopkins snorted in disdain. "So say you. With all your heads put together you could think of no solution. Yet a dolt of a smith displayed more wisdom than your witless Elders and saved the day with a jackscrew. From such stupid tutors as they are, may the Lord preserve us."

John Carver was pale with suppressed anger. "Your remarks are unwarranted, Mr. Hopkins. You are wayward and mutinous as are many of the London people. You have nothing at heart but your own selfish wants. I pray the Lord may show you the error of your ways."

"And may He do likewise for you," he retorted.

The brunt of the pumping was borne by the Leyden men and the mariners. The water stood knee deep in the hold, and it was an arduous task to expel it. At times as the inflow exceeded the outgo we were forced to redouble our exertions, but Captain Jones failed to express any undue alarm. With the mended mainbeam holding fast, little danger awaits us and we can look forward to rounding out our voyage in safety.

Thursday, October 12, 1620

Storms! Tempests! Gales! Is there no mercy in the elements, no halt to their displeasure? Eleven days have passed in which we had but one of fair weather. There is no relief from the assaults of the wind, rain and sea; they will not cease to harry us. Night and day we must man the pumps to keep the ship afloat. The water in the hold has almost reached to our waists, and if it rises much higher we will be driven from the pumps and all will be lost.

The people are worn to wan images of their former selves and move about like gaunt, hollow specters. Weakened as they are by constant exposure to inclement weather, many have become afflicted with coughs and sundry lung ailments. Our cabins reek of filth and stink of human bodies pestering like swine in pigsties. May the Lord have mercy on us. If the storms do not abate we will all be bags of skin and bones or dead ones.

Tomorrow is Friday the 13th, an evil, ill-omened day pledged to misfortune and likely to be fruitful in mishaps and misadventure. An uncanny foreboding has beset me, but I shall be wary and on the alert. Forewarned is forearmed.

Friday, October 27, 1620

Friday the 13th is a fortnight past, and despite my foreboding and caution I can give thanks to the Lord that I live to record the dread misadventure of that evil day. It is a great wonder that I escaped from the sea wherein I now would have been dismembered and gorged in the maws of fishes.

The day (Friday the 13th) was stormy and filled with strong winds and high seas. The ship was stripped of sail and given over to the humor of the tempest. I feared to stir from my cabin, but past midday a familiar of the devil beset and cozened me to go on deck. I had neither ryhme nor reason so to do and my will said "Nay". Yet such was the power of the evil one that my pliant feet bore my resisting body on deck in the midst of the seething elements.

I had hardly taken more than a step or two when a huge wave like a cataract swept aboard and knocked my feet from under me. The pitching of the ship cast me into the sea and down I went fathoms under water and choked with brine. I struggled to the surface and gasped for air. Thinking my end had come, I intrusted my soul to the Lord, when lo! There within arm's reach a length of the topsail halyard was trailing in the sea. If, as it is said, a drowning man grasps at a straw, all the more eagerly I clutched at this firmer link to life.

There have been many rides which history has recorded, but there was never a ride like mine. For did ever a rider have so strange a steed, so watery a chariot and so slender a rein? Yea, and it was a race with the specter of death riding abreast of me. The stakes were life against death. When my grip weakened he stretched forth his bony claws to seize me; when my hold tightened he withdrew disconcerted.

I do not know how long I was dragged through the sea. Numbed with cold and strangled by the brackish water, yet I held the rope clenched between my teeth and entwined my feet about it. Yea, and such was my dread of a watery grave, I verily believe I would have clung to the rope till the *Mayflower* arrived at America. This, praised be the Lord, was not requisite. Some of the mariners had observed the manner in which I had been cast into the sea and they hauled the rope to the ship's edge and got me aboard with boathooks.

"He lives," cried one of the seamen. "It's a miracle that he escaped death."

"He's not saved yet," said another. "He's swallowed half the water in the sea. Below with him, quick."

The world went dark before my eyes and I was in a void space. It seemed that I lay on the bed of the ocean with the *Mayflower* resting on me. The ship's keel was pressing down with its tremendous weight. My chest and ribs were being compressed against my backbone and the blood was forced spurting through my mouth and nose. I grappled with the great hulk to push it off my body, but it was futile. The monstrous vise held me fast and I could not pry myself loose.

Consciousness returned to me. I was in my cabin, encompassed by a ring of anxious, staring eyes. Dr. Fuller was bent over me, kneading my chest vigorously to expel the water from my lungs. The pain in my chest and ribs was one of sheer agony, and I made a feeble effort to ward off his hands.

"Easy, lad, easy," he said softly. "You're bloated with water that's got to be tapped out of you. I'll be as gentle as I can."

He worked for a time with tireless energy. "There," he finally said. "I'll warrant there's not much of the water left in you. Now you'd best go to sleep and get some rest. You'll feel like a new man when you awake."

My head was drowsy and I needed little urging from him. Before my eyes closed in slumber I heard Elizabeth's tearful voice, asking: "Will he live, Dr. Fuller?"

"Will he live? Ha!" he scoffed. "It would take more than such a trifle to do away with him. He'll be well enough before long to lead you to the altar. Never fear for that, my maid."

I was none the worse for the mishap, but death, being a harsh gamester and a sorry loser, was not to be filched of his prey thus lightly. A heavy cold set in, and my lungs were tainted and became so inflamed that I could hardly draw breath. Despite Dr. Fuller's skill it was thought I would perish and that I had been drawn from one watery grave only to be cast into another.

During the past fortnight I hovered at the door to eternity with my life suspended by a hair. No pains were spared in my behalf by Dr. Fuller. Every safeguard at his command was put into play to halt the inroads of the affliction. My own sturdy vitality also aided me in my struggle for survival. Yet if it had not been for the loving care of Elizabeth and the considerate attention of Will Butten, both of whom wore themselves to the bone in my service, I would not have lived through the illness.

Saturday, October 28, 1620

This morning I awoke feeling much better, though still in a weakened state by reason of the ordeal I had undergone. My lungs were tender and my breath came in gasps like that of a fish out of its element. The lengthy confinement had aroused within me an aversion for the dank cabin with its moldy atmosphere. It was murky at all times. No sunlight ever penetrated except at noonday when a few stray beams would be reflected in through the hatchway.

Dr. Fuller came and commented approvingly on my condition. "I fear I'll not have you for a patient much longer. Another week and you'll be as fit as you ever were."

"Another week?" I exclaimed in dismay. "Need I lie here in the cabin all that time? I'm tired of being cooped in below. It retards my recovery. I'd do better if I were able to go above for a while."

"If it warms up you may go on deck later for a half hour or so. But see that you dress warmly and keep clear of the wind. I'll not have you subject yourself to a relapse."

Shortly after midday Will Butten aided me on deck, the first time I had been above since the ill-fated 13th of this month. I sat at the stern to bask in the sun and breathe the brisk air. What a joy it was! I fairly reveled in the invigoration, and new life pulsed through my veins like a stream of elixir. Of all the Lord's blessings to mankind, sunshine and fresh air are accorded the least deference by reason of their abundance; yet if we are deprived of them, their precious qualities become enhanced to exalted heights.

The people gathered around to lavish me with congratulations on my escape from death and to express their joy over my repaired health. I was deeply touched by their show of sentiment. They were strangers to me with reference to blood ties, yet no kith or kin could have displayed more earnest affection and concern for my welfare. Truly the travail of common adversity will often unite mortals in bonds far more enduring than haphazard relationships entailed by reason of birth.

"The Lord in His infinite mercy has seen fit to spare you from the sea and the affliction which followed," remarked John Carver. "So may His blessing guard you through all the years of your life. I am led to believe that you are destined to become a bulwark of our commonwealth, and fate surely must hold great honor in store for you. We older ones will not survive long. The time is almost at hand for many of us. Yet when we are called, it will be a great comfort to know that the brunt of our unfinished labor will be left in the able charge of stalwarts such as you."

I colored deeply at his high-sounding praise and replied that I had done nothing to merit it.

"Nothing to merit it?" cried Stephen Hopkins. "Only listen to him, if you will. By divine intervention he's plucked out of the sea and survives a deathbed illness. Throughout the entire voyage he's displayed a courage and fortitude that's endeared him to all our hearts. He's been dutiful to his superiors, cheerful in the face of discouragement and never shirked or quibbled. Withal he's chary of praise and the very essence of modesty."

"More's the pity others are not governed by his example," observed John Carver with a subtle glance at Stephen Hopkins.

The shaft did not wander astray.

"If that was intended for me, it's not in point," cried Stephen Hopkins flaring up. "And furthermore it's not well taken. No man can say I ever flouted lawful authority in the face. In London my name was ever above reproach. It stood as a byword for obedience and submission to all officers of state. As for my conduct here at sea, it also will withstand scrutiny, if viewed in the light of reason and not prejudice. Your insult is highly out of place, Mr. Carver."

"This is not the time for turmoil," he replied as he fixed his gaze remotely westward.

"True, but if you must air your slurs in public, I'll not suffer them to go unanswered. You hold your peace and I'll do likewise. But you'll not have the last word with me;

at least not while I've a tongue that's able to wag in my mouth."

Happily the dispute was nipped by the timely approach of Captain Jones with two of his mates.

"How now, lad," cried the captain in a jovial humor. "How goes it with you?"

"Much better, thank you," I responded. "It would please me greatly if I could express my gratitude to your men. Their being on the alert was the means of saving my life. I'll be eternally indebted to them."

"Say no more about it," he said, with a wave of the hand. "Getting you out of the water was mere child's play. Though they did maintain you were the strangest breed of fish they ever hauled from the sea. It was a rare catch indeed."

A sally of laughter went up, and he continued: "The way you clung to that rope was little short of heroic. Not many a man would have lived to tell the tale, yet here you are to bear witness to how you outsmarted Father Neptune. How he must be chafing at your escape. You'd better not tempt him that way again. He's known to have a long memory for those who've flaunted him."

"You may rest easy on that score, captain," I answered. "It will be many a day before I'll be able to look the sea in the face without shuddering at the thought of what might have been. But may I ask how long it will be before we're likely to arrive at haven?"

"We've had fair weather while you were confined below and the ship has made moderately good speed. I'll warrant we'll sight land within a week to a fortnight at the most."

His declaration evoked a round of cheers and a hum of animated discourse.

"Hear, hear! A week to a fortnight."

"Captain Jones just averred it."

"We'll be secure in haven."

"A week to a fortnight at the most."

Yet for all I can see there is naught but the boundless ocean at every quarter and land seems a thousand leagues distant.

Sunday, October 29, 1620

The time spent on deck yesterday had wrought a marvel with my condition. In addition thereto I had passed a restful night, and I arose this morning feeling refreshed and in the glow of good health. John Alden was sleeping soundly, but Will Butten was awake, clearing his nose vigorously. His eyes were red as though from irritation and swam in a constant discharge of tear matter.

"What ails you, Will?" I asked in alarm.

"It's only a slight attack of the rheum," he replied. "It's sure to clear up before the day is over."

"You'd best see Dr. Fuller," I advised. "He'll give you something to check it before it becomes grave."

"I'll attend to it myself," he said testily. "I'd be a poor physician's apprentice if I couldn't do that much. Have you heard the news?"

"What news?" I demanded.

"The London men met secretly in the ship's hold last night. None were admitted except Stephen Hopkins' followers."

"And what took place?"

"For one thing they chose him to be their chief."

"There was no need to do that in secret," I said. "He's been their leader since we left Plymouth."

"True, but they went far beyond that. They've declared themselves to be a separate and distinct entity from us and will only abide by such regulations as they deem proper. It's said they'll not join with us in prayer services today and henceforth. This will signal their cleavage from our Company."

It was appalling news indeed, and struck me blank. Not that it was unlooked for, since it had been brewing almost from the hour we had first weighed anchor and set sail on our voyage. Nonetheless it came like a blow in the dark that is anticipated but cannot be evaded.

"Is it a certainty then?" I inquired. "Have they come out with it and made their intentions known?"

"Not entirely," he answered. "A good deal of what I've related is mere rumor and conjecture. We'll see whether or not they appear for services. As for the rest, they may bide their time to await a more auspicious moment before making their avowals open."

"If it is true it will be a bitter pill. What will the Elders do?"

"I don't know. They met in Mr. Carver's cabin till past midnight, but their decision has not been made public. I wish it were in my power to heal the rift. If it could be effected, no price would be too dear to pay."

I hurriedly dressed myself while digesting the evil tidings and rapped on Stephen Hopkins' door.

"Come in," he called.

I entered the cabin and found him alone in bed. In as

calm a voice as I could muster, I said: "It's nearly time for prayer services, Mr. Hopkins. Are you coming?"

He sat up, placed his hands in the region of his midriff and emitted a dubious moan. "I cannot go, lad," he replied, contorting his features in a doleful expression. "I've developed a sudden indisposition of the entrails. They're twisted into a knot the devil couldn't unravel. Make it known to Mr. Brewster, if you will, and present my apologies. I regret I'm unable to appear in person."

"Then the other London people will attend the services?" I asked, feeling somewhat relieved.

His shoulders hunched in an eloquent gesture. "How can I answer for them? I speak for Stephen Hopkins. All others are at liberty to do likewise for themselves."

My face fell as I saw the meaning back of his words, and I observed him scanning me shrewdly.

"Now don't be unduly alarmed," he continued in a soothing voice. "There's no reason for it so far as you're concerned. No doubt you have an inkling of what's in the wind, but you stand high in my favor and I'll see to it that you're not neglected. The London people want me to be their governor. For my part I have no reason to take issue with their choice. A few days' sail distance a virgin land awaits us. I all but hold it in the hollow of my hand. I need only close my fingers on it, and it can be mine to rule for the rest of my days."

He had risen to his feet with his clenched palm outstretched, his eyes aglow with strange fires of desire.

"It's wrong!" I cried in an outburst of anxiety. "Our voyage was undertaken to establish a commonwealth to be ruled by God and not by man. You create dissension and discord. It will lead to strife and mortal injury to all our Company."

"You're but a boy," he remarked, giving me a pitying glance. "You're not versed in the ways of the world. Some day you'll learn that man rises to power by taking a firm hold of his opportunity and making the most of it. If in so doing he must trample certain of his fellowmen underfoot, then more's the pity; yet one cannot be too squeamish about it. We live in a harsh world, and we either rise or fall as we guide ourselves by its standards. You're but a boy," he repeated, "but I'll take you in hand and mold you into stern manhood. You'll shed your fledgling feathers fast enough and become a full-grown bird of prey. And mark what I say at this moment— The time will come when you'll acknowledge I'm right and humbly thank me for having made myself your benefactor."

Brusquely interrupting my storm of protest, he waved me out, saying: "Now don't vex me unduly, for I'm not to be balked by you or anyone else. Go convey my message to Mr. Brewster. And hearken, lad," he added significantly. "I'll not seek to compel you to throw your lot in with me, but I've reposed my confidence in you. See that you don't betray it."

The Sabbath Day services were conducted without the London people. It was a mournful gathering of men and women who see their lives' labor and harvest barren of fruition. Visages seared with care bespoke the troubled spirits that had conceived their grimness. Elder Brewster pleaded zealously for the Lord to restore unity to our severed ranks. And when he gave thanks to Him for my recovery, none said "Amen" with greater fervency than I—unless it was Elizabeth.

Monday, October 30, 1620

Will Butten had coughed intermittently during the night. It was a dry, rasping cough that convulsed his frame. This morning his features were drawn and haggard. I brought water for his parched lips and placed my hand on his forehead. It was burning intensely with fever.

"Did you see Dr. Fuller yesterday?" I asked.

He shook his head.

"You should have done so," I said reprovingly. "There's no telling what might develop from this."

I hastened to Dr. Fuller, and within a few minutes he came bustling into our cabin with mock severity.

"What's this I hear?" he demanded. "My own apprentice taken sick abed? It's a reflection on me. It discredits my profession and I'll not put up with it. Come now, lad, what ails you?"

"Oh, it's nothing to worry about," Will replied.

Dr. Fuller bent over him and felt his brow. "Fever and a cold. A heavy cold, too," he mused. "Why didn't you call me sooner? This is no idle matter."

"I didn't think a cold was worthy of your attention," muttered Will.

"What! Not deserving of my attention?" Dr. Fuller's ire was aroused and mounting higher. "No ailment is too slight to go unheeded. You've been grossly negligent, Will. You hope to be a physician yourself some day, yet you've discarded a major principle of your future calling. Never neglect a minor affliction, or it might spread into a major one and then it may be too late to save the patient. You should have called it to my attention without undue delay."

He glowered at Will and then said, more kindly: "You needn't take my rebuke to heart, but hereafter bear in mind that every deathbed illness has a trifling inception of some sort or other. Don't be alarmed," he quickly interposed as Will's pallor deepened. "You're not seriously ill, and I'll have you up at an early day. But you should have called me sooner. I'll bring you a potion to allay the fever and some medicine for your cold. I'll be back shortly."

I followed him out into the passageway and asked: "He'll get better, will he not, Dr. Fuller?"

He emitted a short laugh. "Of course he will. He's in a weakened state from having played the nursemaid to you during your illness. But there's little to be feared. You may rest assured he'll recover."

The worried look in his eyes belied the promise of his words. I was smitten with pangs of conscience, and heavy hearted, I went back to the cabin to await his return. Nearly a half hour passed before he appeared and accounted for the delay by saying: "I was forced to call on another patient. The maid Elizabeth is ill."

I rose to my feet with a question spurting to my lips: "Not my Elizabeth?"

He nodded in confirmation.

"What ails her?" I asked weakly.

"Also a cold, only a lighter one than Will's. She'll be better before long. There's no worry with her."

"I'll return soon," I said, and rushed off to her.

She was lying in bed swathed in covers and sorely stricken with a malignant attack of the rheum. Its inroads seemed to have wasted her sadly; she appeared a mere shadow of her former likeness. A nameless dread shackled my tongue and I could say nothing.

"John," she gently said, "don't stare at me as if you fear the worst will come to pass. I'll be rid of this cold in a short time."

"The Lord grant it be so," I responded in a somber vein.

"Dr. Fuller says Will Butten is sick," she went on. "Is he any better?"

"I can't say. He's assured me that Will and you are certain to recover. This is an evil day that you both were taken sick."

"But an evil day precedes a fairer morrow. So take heart and don't be so depressed."

Put to shame by her courage, I remarked: "One would think I'm the sick one instead of you. I'm a poor visitor for a sickbed."

"What does it matter? If I'm in good spirits, then

there's all the more reason to believe it won't be too long before I recover."

I lingered a time before leaving for my cabin to see how Will fared. He was asleep, and Dr. Fuller motioned for me to be silent.

"He's somewhat better," he whispered. "By the time he awakes the fever should be gone. Keep an eye on him and call me as soon as he's up."

I passed the day hurrying back and forth from one sickbed to the other. Will awoke a few hours after noonday and I advised Dr. Fuller of it. He came back with me to test Will's brow and feel his pulse.

"Greatly improved," he announced with evident satisfaction. "The fever is almost abated and the pulse has slowed down. You'll be well in a day or two. You can count on it, Will."

"What about Elizabeth?" I inquired.

"You need have no fear for her. In good truth I'll warrant they'll both make a rapid recovery."

Yet despite Dr. Fuller's conviction, my heart sorely misgives me and I commit them both to the tender mercy of the Lord.

Tuesday, October 31, 1620

This morning Will seemed fairly better. Dr. Fuller called early and evidently was in an ill humor and all out of sorts.

"No fever and your pulse is back to normal," he told Will. "Another day or two of rest, and if you're in bed after then it will be for the reason that you're outright lazy. So look lively and don't impose overlong on my easy disposition."

"Never fear for that," said Will. "I'll be thankful enough to get up. You'll not find me in bed the moment after you say the word."

"How is Elizabeth?" I asked.

Dr. Fuller looked at me with an expression of ill-concealed annoyance.

"You are exceedingly wearing," he complained. "A thousand times a day I hear nothing from you except 'How is Elizabeth?' If it's any comfort to you, she's well, very well indeed. But I myself am getting most unwell from your harassing me. I pray she may recover quickly before you drive me to my own sickbed. Your inquiries cause me more distraction than a pesthouse full of sick."

He snorted in disdain and Will snickered at my discomfort. There was a timid knock at the door.

"See who it is," said Dr. Fuller to me. "For all I know it may be the maid herself, and you can ask her how she is to your heart's content. Only leave me in peace."

It was William Mullins' daughter, Priscilla.

"Is John awake?" she shyly inquired.

I knew whom she meant, but being nettled by Dr. Fuller's ridicule, I answered crossly: "John? What John?"

"How many Johns are there?" she demanded.

"I don't know. My name is also John."

"You're not the John I want. I mean John Alden."

"You may have your precious John," Dr. Fuller called to her. "See how peacefully he sleeps. He snores so gently the ship heaves with his every breath."

She stamped her foot and cried: "It's not so. But I've heard it said, Dr. Fuller, that you snore loud enough to bring your dead patients back to life. Is it true?"

She gazed at him with feigned innocence, an arch smile playing at her lips.

"The pox seize her," he muttered under his breath. "John," he said to me, "arouse the sleeping Adonis and say that his ladylove impatiently awaits him. It's a pretty kettle of fish with these young lovers," he went on mumbling. "No deference for grey hairs or anything else. Speak jestingly of one and the other flies in your face."

John Alden was stirring in bed, and I imparted the news to him.

"Tell her I'll be on deck presently," he said, all aflustered.

"Tell her yourself," I tartly answered.

"Tell her, lad, tell her," pleaded Dr. Fuller. "Or else she'll linger at the door and pester us with more of her impudence. Tell her, and good riddance."

She departed after I delivered the message. John Alden hurriedly dressed, and after a brief inquiry as to Will's health he hastened off.

"There he goes," observed Dr. Fuller. "The tongueless lover. He's quite fond of her and it's an open book that she's enamoured with him. She's waiting for him to say that which her heart yearns to hear. But dolt that he is, for all his good graces and fair speech, when he's with her he blushes and stammers uncouth words which a boor would not confess to be his own. Love is indeed a great mystery. I freely acknowledge it's beyond the bounds of my comprehension."

"It doesn't seem likely that he'll return to England when his time runs out," I remarked.

"It certainly does not," responded Dr. Fuller. "At least not without her. He's enmeshed in that from which his time will never run out. I for one am well pleased with it, for he's a likely youth and we'll have good need of him. She's too pert and forward, but she'll make him a good wife. That is if she ever succeeds in placing the halter about his neck."

With Will and Elizabeth on the road to recovery, my thoughts drifted to other channels. This was the last day of October. The nights have been getting colder and each morning the air is chilled by the breath of the north wind. Winter was close at hand with no land in sight. The *Mayflower's* speed has been retarded by reason of the fact that Captain Jones fears to overpress her with sail; to do so would give rise to the danger of straining her hull. However, he maintains we should reach our haven in little more than a week.

Then there is the trouble with the London people. Each day they wax more arrogant. Rumors both whispered and aloud are flying in furious outbursts of conjecture. It is said that as soon as land is sighted they stand prepared to seize the ship and deal with us in a high-handed manner. The Leyden people are to be dropped off at the first landing-place while they propose to sail on and find a more suitable habitation for themselves. Even further, some say it is their intention to make bondslaves of the Leyden people.

No one knows with certainty how much truth lies in these rumors. The weight of opinion is to the effect that they are highly colored. As for myself, I dread the approaching cleavage as a sufficient evil in itself. Stephen Hopkins is greedy for power and will leave no stone unturned to attain his end, let it cost what it may. Unless he is halted in his evil plan, the Lord only knows what the outcome will be, and He alone can forestall it.

Wednesday, November 1, 1620

One way or another John Billington is ever astew in a
pot of mischief of his own brewing. He had been gaming
with the seamen during the entire passage and his good
fortune or skill was such that he had gleaned them as
clean as whistles, even to the shirts on their backs. Indeed
many of them had been forced to give him bond to their
wages earned on the voyage.

Today in the forenoon I was on deck for a breath of
air. A hubbub broke loose in the forecastle and Billington,
all battered and bleeding, dashed out. At his heels were
half a score seamen yelling like so many fiends and furies.
With his tattered garments flapping in the wind, he scurried along like a hare before the hounds and cut so sorry
a figure I could scarcely contain myself for mirth. Down
the hatchway he tumbled with his pursuers after him.

I joined the fringe of the hue and cry which came to a
halt at Stephen Hopkins' cabin. The seamen were pounding at the door and shouting abusively for Billington to
show himself.

"Out with you, you thief."

"Come out, you cheat, you swindler."

"We'll have your life's blood for this."

A flood of oaths and curses was profusely intermingled
with their outcries.

The door swung open and Stephen Hopkins appeared, armed with a musket.

"Stand back, you wolves," he cried. "What's the meaning of this outrage? Stand back or I'll shoot, I warn you. Go no further; I'm not a man to be trifled with. Ha, Ned Dotey," he called, with a backward glance. "Have the other musket ready for me as quick as I discharge this one."

The seamen recoiled from the formidable front he presented.

"We've no quarrel with you, Mr. Hopkins," said one. "It's John Billington we want. He's been cheating and must make us satisfaction."

"It's a slanderous falsehood," answered Stephen Hopkins. "John Billington is an honorable man and I'll vouch for him by all that's holy. You're envious because he's won from you. Gamesters should accept their losses as cheerfully as their winnings, but instead you come crying like children who've been deprived of their sweets. Captain Jones shall hear from me on this. Now be on your way with the pack of you, you sulky dogs."

"We caught him swindling us and we'll not be denied," growled another seaman. "He'll make us satisfaction or we'll have our vengeance. We'll return armed to the teeth and take him by force if need be."

"Hold a while," exclaimed Stephen Hopkins in alarm as they started withdrawing. He then called: "John Billington, step forward and face your accusers. If you're in the right you'll have nothing to fear, and if you're wrong we'll find a peaceful remedy. Come forward, I say."

Cringing in terror Billington appeared at the side of his protector.

"Now by your leave," said Stephen Hopkins to the seamen, "I'll act the magistrate to decide who's in the right and what's to be done. Are you willing?"

"We're not willing," declared the spokesman. "You're in his favor."

"Here and now I take a solemn oath to judge you both impartially," he declared. "If I allow any prejudice to sway my judgment, may the Lord strike me dead before your eyes. Does that satisfy you?"

"Aye, it does, Mr. Hopkins. We'll abide by your judgment. We trapped Billington cheating us at cards. He's been doing it since the first day we started gaming with him."

"What proof have you to sustain this charge?"

"We suspected he's a sleight-of-hand wizard who can draw cards out of the thin air. Today we trapped him. He overstepped himself and held two knaves of spades, each of them as black a knave as he himself is. All men know there's but one to a pack, yet he held two."

"What have you to say to this?" Stephen Hopkins sternly demanded of Billington.

"I've been upright with them, I swear it," he cried. "The two knaves were dealt me after the cards had been shuffled. I don't know how it happened."

"You know well enough," said one of the seamen scornfully. "You plucked the second one from your sleeve or breeches."

"I did not," he protested. "You accuse me most unjustly. The Lord will bear me out."

"If He doesn't, we will. We'll bear you out into the sea."

Ominous mutterings went up from the seamen, and Stephen Hopkins was quick to sense the peril.

"Now, Billington," he said aloud for all to hear. "It may be true that you're unjustly accused and the seamen are in error—"

"We're not," they chorused.

"Don't be so hasty," he pleaded. "I was about to say to him, what if he does forfeit the few paltry pounds he's won from you? Friendship and good fellowship are far more priceless than base material wealth. If your friendships hang in the balance, then I say let him give up his gains and keep your esteem. He'll be the richer by it and so will you. John Billington, my decree is that you make the seamen satisfaction for all you've won from them. Do you agree?"

Billington squirmed and swallowed hard, but said: "If you wish it, Mr. Hopkins, I'll do so to please you."

"It is my wish and will please me well. How now, men? Does my judgment meet with your approval?"

A loud cheer resounded, and Stephen Hopkins called: "Ned, Ned Dotey. Come out and serve drinks for the seamen. I've never had the pleasure of mingling with a more worthy crew."

I could not help but admire the masterful way in which Stephen Hopkins had veered a near misfortune into a pleasant outcome. He had started by calling the seamen "wolves" and "sulky dogs" and ended by wheedling them into the belief that they were the salt of the earth. They had come with blood in their eyes and curses on their lips, and left singing his praises for all to hear. Plainly he is a man to be reckoned with. What a relief it would be if he were only aligned with us!

In the evening Will complained of weariness. "My limbs are so weak they feel as if they were dead weight," he remarked to me. "I don't know what it is. Up till sundown my full strength had almost returned, but now it seems to have ebbed away."

"It's likely you're tired and in need of rest," I suggested. "Is there something I can do for you? Perhaps I ought to call Dr. Fuller."

He mournfully shook his head. "It would do no good to call him. I fear no one can help me except the Lord."

"Will!" I cried in anxiety. "What do you mean?"

"Nothing. Simply that the Lord will help me," he replied, with a brave smile. "I'll feel better by morning. Go to sleep, John, and don't fret over me."

My heart a lump of ice, I went to bed with a fervent prayer for him on my lips. The Lord grant he is better by morning, yet I look for the worst.

Thursday, November 2, 1620

My fears were borne out with a vengeance. This morning Will's appearance was startling in the extreme. His features were so wan and pinched they seemed to have shrunk into his countenance. A sickly pallor had overspread all vestige of color. It was as grisly a hue as that of death itself. Only the rise and fall of his breast and the dully lighted eyes gave evidence of life in him.

"How do you feel, Will?" I asked with bated breath.

Without moving or glancing at me, he replied: "I'm weaker. There's no strength left. John, I'll never recover. I'm coming to my end. I know it."

The echo of despair in his feeble voice sent a shudder through me. I rushed at top speed to Dr. Fuller's cabin and pounded on the door, calling aloud for him.

"Who's there?" he demanded from within. "What's up?"

"Come quickly," I cried. "Will is in a desperate state. He says he's coming to his end."

"I'll be there at once."

I dashed back to the cabin and said to Will: "Keep up your courage. Dr. Fuller will soon be here to help you."

"It's useless," he answered in a listless tone. "He can do nothing to save me."

The savor from his breath was highly offensive. It

forced me to turn my head away from him as I said: "Don't speak that way, Will. Dr. Fuller is sure to make you well again."

Dr. Fuller entered with an assumed air of cheerfulness. "Ha, what's this? My patient has had a relapse? It's nothing. All have it before the final recovery. You'll be better soon. Never fear for that."

"I'll not get better," responded Will. "I'd as soon have it over with. I have no fear of death. I'll welcome it."

"Stop your prattling," Dr. Fuller sternly ordered. "Rid your mind of these foolish notions. I say you'll recover, and I ought to know. Open your mouth and let me see your tongue."

He peered at the organ and pressed his fingers into the gums about Will's teeth. "Do you hunger for food?" he asked. "Would you eat something that had a relish for you?"

Will's features twisted wryly. "I have no stomach for food. I can't eat. It would be distasteful to me."

"You must eat. How else will you regain your strength? Go ask Mrs. Carver if she'll prepare some broth," he directed me, adding in a whisper: "Perhaps she can throw in something in the way of greens."

Mrs. Carver had no greens, but said she would use dried peas and onions. I informed Dr. Fuller of this.

"Greens would serve the purpose far better," he muttered, with a dubious shake of the head. "But it may be the peas and onions will do."

When the broth was brought he fed it forcibly to Will who evinced a great aversion for it. After swallowing a few spoonfuls he pushed it away and could not be swayed to partake of more. Dr. Fuller cajoled and threatened, but to no avail. Will's vigor was in so meager a state that the slight exertion involved in eating had sapped his strength to exhaustion. He panted for air and then fell asleep.

"The poor lad," muttered Dr. Fuller with a break in his voice. "To be afflicted with so dire a malady."

"What ails him?" I inquired.

Dr. Fuller's voice fell to a horrified whisper. "He has the symptoms of scurvy. If it's a forerunner of this scourge, then others aboard ship may become afflicted. May the good Lord have mercy on him and also on us."

My heart fell at the mention of this accursed sickness so frequently encountered on lengthy sea voyages. "Are you sure of it, Dr. Fuller?"

"Not quite. There's still some doubt in my mind. He has a weakened body, sallow features, softened gums and a swollen tongue. These are the indications of scurvy. Also, you see how he's depressed in spirit? He knows he'll not get better, he's ready to welcome death. That's another symptom, though like the others it's common to sundry ailments. We must keep up his spirit. If he loses the will to survive, then the battle is lost before it's even begun."

"Is there no cure?" I asked.

"There's no known medicine for this purpose," he

answered. "The affliction comes from partaking of stale, unvaried victuals. Fresh meat and greens would be likely to effect a cure, but our store is exhausted. In all probabilities he'll live till we reach land and then we may get what we need for him. At least there's no immediate danger, so let's keep our hopes high."

This was far easier said than done. With Will in such a doleful plight I could hardly restrain my distress, yet I endeavored to abide by Dr. Fuller's counsel with a semblance of outward cheer. I kept a close vigil and would not stir from the cabin. To the many inquiries of the people, I replied that he had undergone a minor relapse, but it was not of grave concern. Nor would I allow them to view his stricken countenance, saying Dr. Fuller had forbidden his being disturbed.

He awoke near noonday with his condition neither better nor worse, except that his pulse beat had quickened. I could not prevail on him to eat the broth. His stomach had not come to him, and the mere sight of food was so revolting to his innards that he was seized with violent retchings. Dr. Fuller purged him and then fed him a small portion despite his feeble protests. The task was an odious one. It inspired me with an aversion for a physician's calling.

I think this was the longest and dreariest day ever spent aboard ship, not excepting those days when I had been confined abed. It seemed as if darkness would never fall. With the oncoming of night Will displayed a degree of improvement. It was also a comfort that Dr. Fuller pronounced Elizabeth cured of her cold and withdrew all restrictions entailed by her illness. Thus the Lord tempers evil with good; but if it were not a blasphemy to say it, the pity is that good does not come without evil.

Friday, November 3, 1620

This morning Will's condition was markedly better. His eyes shone with a renewed luster and a faint bloom of color had mounted to his cheeks. What was even more noteworthy, his hunger irked him into clamoring for food. Yesterday's broth had soured and Mrs. Carver prepared some afresh for him. He devoured it avidly to the last drop, giving every indication of having relished the repast. With these auspicious omens, Dr. Fuller and I could hardly contain our exultation.

"The tide's turned in your favor," Dr. Fuller gleefully announced. "I predicted you'd be on the road to recovery. What's a small ailment to sturdy young blood like yours? A mere pin, less than nothing. Now speak truthfully, lad— Don't you feel as though your infirmities were fleeing from you?"

"I do feel much better," acknowledged Will with more animation than he had heretofore shown. "How soon will it be before I recover?"

"Now don't be too hasty," Dr. Fuller warily cautioned. "It may take a few weeks, but that's of no importance. What counts is that you're getting better. Meanwhile be of good cheer and hold your impatience in check."

I hurried off to impart the joyful tidings to Elizabeth.

Our hearts were aglow with contentment, but not for long. Will's malady is a specter beclouding our joy. He took a turn for the worse after sundown. His pallor deepened and his pulse quickened to an alarming speed. He panted in short, jerky breaths as if his lungs were choked. All signs of good health vanished and his depression of spirits returned with tenfold volume.

Dr. Fuller uncovered him and scanned his body. His ankles and lower limbs were thickly covered with ash-pale spots as if the flesh had been pinched or bruised. Dr. Fuller stooped and made his examination with studied care. He was silent, but his pensive brow betrayed the anxiety stirred into being by the appearance of these telltale marks.

"There's nothing to be feared," he finally declared. "You must not lose faith. Keep your courage high and don't yield to your misgivings. That's the medicine I'm prescribing for you."

There was no response from Will.

Dr. Fuller motioned for me to step out of the cabin. "He's clutched in the final stages of scurvy," he whispered. "The spots on his limbs foretell it. Our one hope is to reach land where we might get some fresh meat and greens for him. There's no other remedy. The ship creeps along at a snail's pace. Ask Captain Jones if he can increase her speed. Tell him it's most urgent."

I encountered the captain on deck and made known to him the imperative need for haste.

He shook his head dubiously as he said: "It would be a hazard to overpress the ship with sail. Our present speed should bring us to land within a week. Will he hold out till then?"

"Every hour is precious," I answered. "A day's sail shortened may be the means of saving him from death."

"With a life at stake I must run the risk. I trust it will be to a good purpose. We'll clap on all sail the ship can bear."

He called his mates and gave orders accordingly. They expressed astonishment and called attention to the danger of this course, but he cut them short with a stern warning that he was the master of the ship and in no need of counsel from them.

The seamen went aloft in the twilight and unfurled the topsails to the wind. For a moment the *Mayflower* quivered under the stress of added pressure; then she forged ahead by leaps and bounds. It was as if she sensed the approaching enactment of a tragedy and gave promise of exerting herself to the utmost to prevent its fulfillment.

Saturday, November 4, 1620

With death flying hard in our wake, the *Mayflower*
swooped westward on the wings of the wind, shearing
league after league from the distance between us and our
haven. Land is to be sighted any day, and the people are
restless in their yearning to see the voyage ended. And
now we reaped the harvest, bitter as gall, from the seeds
of discord sowed and nurtured by John Billington. Our
Company has been rent asunder by factions. The London
men, captained by Stephen Hopkins and irked on by
Billington, have flung aside all pretense of unity and are
in open mutiny.

The rupture occurred on deck past midday. Most of
the Leyden people were assembled at the bow, gazing
eagerly across the expanse of water as if expecting to see
land rise up out of the sea. Suddenly the London men
came up the hatchway in a body and trooped across the
deck with a semblance of military formation, though not
bearing arms. First came Stephen Hopkins strutting with
a lordly air. Flanking him were John Billington and Edward Dotey, followed in pairs by John Rigdale, Solomon
Prower, Edward Leister, John Langermore and others,
tallying nearly a full score in all. But I could not see a
single Leyden man in their ranks.

We turned inquiringly toward them as they approached, hardly knowing what to expect. When Stephen Hopkins was within some ten paces, he called a halt and advanced with John Billington and Edward Dotey to accost John Carver.

"Mr. Carver, I appear as spokesman in behalf of the London people," he said, raising his voice to be heard by all. "Our voyage is nearing its end and the time has come for us to make known our intentions. We embarked with no thought of any schism between ourselves and your Leyden people. If one has arisen, it's not through any fault of ours. You have ever sought to subject us to indignities. Our grievances have gone unheeded. Again I say this schism has arisen through no fault of ours."

"It surely is no fault of ours either," replied John Carver. "We've made every honest effort to placate the London people. We've agreed to all their reasonable demands. Even now we stand prepared to right any wrongs or affronts to which they may have unwittingly been subjected."

Stephen Hopkins shook his head firmly in denial. "Your offer comes too late, Mr. Carver. The wound has festered too deeply to be healed by fair words and promises. Besides, we Londoners are so widely at variance with your Leyden people that we can never be welded with them into one firm body. We've come to America to find freedom of thought and liberty of movement. Once we've landed we're not to be trampled on or restricted by your laws and regulations. Every man, we say, should be his own judge of what is morally right or wrong, except that he shall not give public offense to his fellowmen. Now you know our minds in the matter."

"That can never be," averred John Carver, speaking with great earnestness. "If every man is to be his own judge of what is morally right or wrong, then there will be no government or rule of justice, but rather of might. Think well, Mr. Hopkins. We are about to seek habitation in a wild and barbarous land. Our numbers are pitifully few, the dangers many. If we hope to escape extinction we must preserve a united front to the enemies we are sure to encounter. All should lay aside their personal animosities and exert themselves to the furtherance of the commonweal."

"We're prepared to join with you in defense against our mutual enemies," declared Stephen Hopkins. "But we'll not abide by your rule or government. The commonweal means little to us. It's a contraption of the weaklings to insure their protection by the stronger ones and to enable them to partake of the fruit of toil by the able-bodied. We'll not hinder you, and all we ask is to go our own way without hindrance from you. The new land is broad enough for both without our treading on each other's toes. Do I make myself clear?"

"Not entirely," said John Carver. "Your intention then is to seek a habitation separate and apart from ours?"

"We'll find a habitation perhaps nearby yours," answered Stephen Hopkins. "But we propose to establish a commonwealth under our own jurisdiction. We'll divide our store of provisions and treat with you as to the terms of each coming to the other's defense in the event either should be attacked by savages. Aside from that we declare ourselves free and clear from you and yours, now and forever after."

John Carver shook his head dolefully. "Nothing but evil will come of your reckless course. We cannot coerce you to stay with us, yet reason must dictate it would be far more discreet if you did. Let us hold fast in one body till we are firmly entrenched in the new land. Then if you wish you may establish yourselves elsewhere. But meanwhile if we divide our forces and provisions we'll be lost. We'll all perish in the wilderness. Heed what I say, Mr. Hopkins."

"Spare yourself these dismal croakings," he curtly responded. "It will avail you nothing. I've stated the express desires of the London people. You have soured their stomachs and they're not to be swayed from their purpose. My advice is that you accept it with a good grace. We hope to be peaceable and friendly toward you, but if you seek to cross us then we'll resort to arms in defense of our liberties. After you've discussed it with your Elders, you can inform me if they'll abide by our terms. All else is of no interest to us."

He faced about and walked off with the London men trailing him. When the last of them had gone down the hatchway, our chief men hastily conferred on how best to cope with the tragic situation. Captain Standish favored seizing Stephen Hopkins and John Billington and putting them in irons as the best means of stifling the revolt. The others feared this might lead to bloodshed and thus be the means of driving deeper the wedge and widening the breach beyond hope of repair.

Out of the diversity of opinion the distracted Elders concluded to speak softly to the Londoners, thinking thereby to bring them into ultimate concord with us. To my mind Captain Standish was right. Soft speech will only embolden the malcontents and spur them into making stronger demands. But the Elders have put their faith in the Lord and look to Him to restore peace and unity in our severed ranks.

Sunday, November 5, 1620

In all likelihood this was our last Sabbath Day at sea and by far the most saddened one. Will Butten is nigh unto death's door. It is even doubted if he will survive the night through. The grim specter of death hovering in the offing is about to claim him for its own and casts its dread shadow over the *Mayflower*. A hushed awe has fallen on the people, a mournful air of dejection which precedes an oncoming misfortune.

Early this morning the flame of life flickered feebly in Will, so feebly that Dr. Fuller gave up all hope for recovery. The physician's eyes were moist and his voice quavered with emotion as he made this heartrending disclosure outside the cabin. A torrent of grief welled up within me and I turned aside to conceal it before going back into the cabin. Dr. Fuller departed to spread the dire news among the people.

They came pressing into the cabin with bowed heads and prayers on their lips, staying but for a few moments to make way for others. Old and young stood muted in sorrow as they gazed on Will's ravaged countenance. None was more deeply affected than the Elder, William Brewster. With his white head bowed low, he sobbed piteously as if his tender heart would be torn in twain, and he prayed long and earnestly at Will's bedside. It would have sufficed to move a stone to tears. I cannot recall it without a moistening of the eyelids.

The people went on deck for prayer services, leaving me alone with Will. My emotions burst all bounds of restraint and convulsed me in the throes of anguish. Will stirred out of his apathy and called to me.

"John, don't weep for me," he whispered. "It can do no good. I'd rather you'd pray for me. Ask Mr. Hopkins if he and the London people will attend the prayer services and do likewise. Tell him it would be of great comfort to me."

Stephen Hopkins was in his cabin with his wife, their youngest child Oceanus, and their oldest, Giles. Mrs. Hopkins' eyes were red from weeping, and he himself was steeped in abject woe.

"You know about Will's condition, Mr. Hopkins?" I asked in a dull voice.

"Only too well," he affirmed with a sad shake of the head. "I feel it too keenly for words. It's moved me to compassion as if he were my own flesh and blood. What a mortal pity that one so young and full of promise should be taken before he's even reached his prime. I'd leave no stone unturned to aid him with all that's in my power. But what good are mere wishes and intentions? All I can do is moan at this misfortune."

"There's something else you can do. He's asked that you attend the prayer services and pray for him."

He glanced searchingly at me. "You're certain he's asked it?"

"This very moment," I replied with conviction. "He said I should tell you it would be of great comfort to him."

"I'll do it if it will comfort him a hair. Come, Bess," he said to his wife. "We'll go on deck and join in prayer for the lad. Who knows? It may be the Lord will be moved to send him succor."

"He also asked that all the London people do likewise," I added, quickly following up my advantage.

A heavy frown furrowed his brow as he meditated briefly. It vanished, and he declared: "And why not? Shall it be said the lad lies on his deathbed and the London people refused to pray for him? Out with petty disputes at a time like this. Giles, tell Ned Dotey he's to spread the word that the London people are to join in the prayer services. Let the Lord see with His own eyes that we're united in prayer for the lad's recovery. Go quickly now."

Thus it was that the Londoners laid aside their enmity and raised their voices together with the Leyden people in prayer for Will Butten. Oh, how Elder Brewster beseeched the Lord that He might spare him unto us. How the aged shepherd pleaded for the blighted lamb of his flock! Yea, his eyes blinded with tears, he supplicated with such fervency that all hearts were touched and none were dry-eyed. And so through the day we prayed for Will.

The oncoming nightfall brought an end to our prayers, but did not abate our manifestations of grief. Tears, tears, bitter tears, there was no end to their flow. And to the stifled sobbing of the womenfolk was added the tearful wailing of children, too young to understand the reason for our lamentations, yet old enough to sense that something was dreadfully amiss.

Monday, November 6, 1620

Will Butten is dead. It hardly seems possible; unbelieving, the mind doubts that which the hand has recorded. I stare about the cabin, my thoughts in utter confusion. It lacks an hour to bedtime. There stands the little bed in which he was wont to sleep, but this night it will be vacant. In a corner is his luggage with the musty tomes in which he so often delved, but nevermore to be scanned by him. Let the eye rove where it will, every object recalls his presence with a prodding and searing of the heart. He is gone from our midst; the first of our Company to be taken by death, but leaving a remembrance that will withstand time's onslaught during the span of our mortal lives.

Two months ago to a day we sailed from Plymouth harbor. Will was in the flush of youthful hope and aspiration; a paragon of uprightness, a pillar of fortitude, an example of oncoming manhood in its best aspects. His earnest yet cheerful mien, his friendly spirit, his eagerness to aid those in distress, his thousand and one goodly qualities and virtues had stamped him as an image of the Lord's own likeness. And now his voice is stilled, his eyes are closed in eternal slumber. Oh, woeful disaster, Will

Butten is dead. Even now his poor body rests leagues astern of us on the bed of the sea, the spot unmarked but not unhallowed, for his death came peacefully in the holy afterglow of the Lord's Day.

Last night his eyes closed as though he had completed his last earthly endeavor and he fell into a stupor. His breathing was slow and labored. Dr. Fuller bent over to hear the heart beat, thinking him to be in the clutch of death. The people cramming the passageway adjoining the cabin waited with bated breath to hear the physician's pronouncement.

"He'll not come out of it," said Dr. Fuller. "I doubt if he'll survive past midnight."

The news was taken up and borne like an eddy from lip to ear. It reached the furthermost people in the passageway. A drawn-out wave of stifled moans and sobs followed in its wake; then fervent prayers went up for the soul soon to wing its way to the great beyond. By midnight Will was still breathing heavily, but with no other sign of life. The people began to disband, except those who intended to keep a vigil over him until the end came.

"You're worn out and badly in need of rest," Dr. Fuller remarked to me. "Go sleep in my cabin for the night. There's nothing you can do here."

"I'd rather stay while there's life in him," I answered. "It may be he'll revive and have some message. I'd never forgive myself if I were not present."

He made no further attempt to dissuade me. In addition to Dr. Fuller, the others who expressed their intention to linger at the deathbed were William Brewster, John Carver and our cabin mate, John Alden.

Time dragged heavily during the night; the only interruptions occurred when divers of the people came gliding into the cabin momentarily and departed after due inquiry. A few hours before daybreak Will aroused himself from his stupor and declared his readiness to consign his soul to the Almighty.

William Brewster, the kindly servant of the Lord, ministered to him with surpassingly hopeful words and prayers. Oh, that one heart, the Elder's, could abound in such earnest tenderness, such heartfelt compassion. Its lavish outpouring swept through the death chamber like a celestial strain of melody and soothed Will into the belief that a far better life awaited him in the hereafter. His eyes lit up with newborn luster, the spirit of godliness shone like a halo about his countenance.

He called me to him and said: "John, the maid I left in Austerfield— Her name is Alice Mayfield. She'll be waiting to hear from me. You'll get word to her that I died with her name on my lips?"

I was too choked to speak. I nodded my head in assent.

He extended his hand, saying: "You do not fear to clasp hands with me?"

I took his feeble, wasted hand and pressed it gently.

"This is the end," he said. "I set off on a voyage to a new land, not thinking to arrive so soon at the Kingdom of Heaven. But so much the better. John, if you can, remember me as a brother who died at sea."

He then said his farewell to William Brewster, calling him "Dearest father," and to Dr. Fuller, John Carver and John Alden. A few minutes later he breathed his last.

This morning at daybreak our Company mournfully assembled on deck in somber attire for the burial. Though the Leyden people are in the custom of interring their dead without benefit of religious services, Elder Brewster stretched a point and delivered a fitting eulogy, taking for his text a passage from the Book of Deuteronomy: "And the Lord said unto him, this is the land * * * : I have caused thee to see it with thine eyes, but thou shalt not go over thither." And as our reverend Elder spoke, his voice broke in grief and anguish; he fell on his knees and the tears poured down his withered cheeks as he wept aloud without restraint.

Oh, what doleful sorrows. What sobs racked every frame, what tears flowed from every eye, what cries were wrung from every heart. It was the saddest sight ever witnessed by mortal man. Yea, Captain Jones and the seamen, weatherbeaten and hardened, could hardly contain their tears. The people of London and those of Leyden sobbed on each other's necks. And shall I ever forget how Stephen Hopkins rocked and moaned in a piteous outburst of woe?

I forbear to say more. There are bounds to human grief that cannot be transgressed, and when the heart is surcharged the overflow helps appease the anguished soul. And so is ended Will Butten with all his earthly hopes and despairs, his joys and sorrows, his griefs and pleasures. May the Lord take his soul into His safekeeping and grant him peace and repose forevermore. Amen.

Tuesday, November 7, 1620

The death of Will Butten, though a sore blow and a grievous wound, was instrumental in restoring peace to our severed ranks and knitting our discordant Company into a firm unity. For in the face of death man sees how pitiful is the struggle that must end in the grave, how futile is life unless it be a godly one, and how debased is the individual who lives only for his own gain and pays no heed to the welfare of his fellowmen. The rank and file of the Londoners were brought to a humble contemplation of their petty waywardness and awaited word from their leader that a concord had been established with the Leyden people.

This was not long in forthcoming. In the forenoon I took the opportunity of calling on Stephen Hopkins.

"How now, Mr. Hopkins?" I inquired. "Are you still determined to keep our people rent in factions?"

"Nay, lad," he answered. "It's been preying heavily on my mind and I'm convinced there must be peace between us and the Leyden people. Come with me, if you will. We'll see Mr. Carver and make it known to him. The sooner done, the better."

At John Carver's cabin, Mrs. Carver excused herself as we entered. Stephen Hopkins returned John Carver's courtly greeting and said to me: "Stand by the door, lad, and let no one enter. There are matters to be discussed that had best be kept from prying ears."

They faced each other in awkward silence for a moment. Then Stephen Hopkins opened the discourse.

"Mr. Carver, to err is a human failing, but to persist in error after one's eyes have been opened is an attribute of a knave or simpleton. Without undue credit to myself, I maintain I'm neither one nor the other. I acknowledge my defaults here in your confidence; but self-esteem does not permit me to do so in public, nor to crave forgiveness from you or anyone else. Let it suffice to say that I've swallowed my pride and come before you as a man who's filled with remorse for his misdeeds, yet asks no sympathy or indulgence."

"Nothing more need be said and no amends need be made," replied John Carver quietly. "All that remains is to make plans for the good and welfare of our people."

"That I'm prepared to do fully," declared Stephen Hopkins. "What has happened is a thing of the past and can't be remedied, but hereafter let there be no more dissension between your people and mine. We're all Englishmen and we'll join forces to labor for the furtherance of our joint interests. I'm prepared to call a truce for all time to come. In the name of the Lord, let us cease wrangling and live in peace and friendship."

I echoed John Carver's fervent "amen," and he said: "Mr. Hopkins, your praiseworthy statements will lift a grave burden from all our shoulders. Civil commotion has brought ruin to flourishing commonwealths and mighty empires. Then how could it do otherwise to a weak settlement such as ours will be, encompassed by the dangers of the wilderness? We must be one compact body, or else there'd be small likelihood of our survival. Furthermore it is not our intention to restrict any with oppressive laws, but to guide ourselves by such reasonable regulations as will affect the common welfare without depriving individuals of their freedom. All shall have equal rights and liberties."

Stephen Hopkins nodded in approval. "That's as it should be. Now how do you propose that the people should be governed?"

"We shall choose a governor to rule in all things civil and a captain to have command in matters military. The governor will be chosen to hold office yearly by the most male voices of twenty-one years of age or over. All his acts and doings shall ever be subject to the approval of the people as a body."

"It meets with my full sanction," said Stephen Hopkins. "But hearken, Mr. Carver, we'd best keep a weather-eye open for John Billington and a few others. He's the main one to fear. He'll do us mischief if he's not held in restraint."

It was intensely gratifying to hear his use of the plurals, "we" and "us" as if he already considered himself aligned against the evil-doers.

Book-of-the-Month Club, Inc., Camp Hill, Pa. 17012

38578

YOUR ACCT. NO.
1324316648   1 MO 273

Dividend Order Form

DIVIDEND CREDIT STATUS   +3

ITEM NUMBER	TITLE	NO. OF COPIES

DIVIDEND ORDERS ONLY

IMPORTANT: If the Book-Dividend you want calls for more credits than you now have—or more than you will acquire as the result of your purchases in the coming month—the system permits immediate shipment of the Book-Dividend ordered. You can make up the shortage by subsequent purchases.

PRINTED IN U.S.A.

"I dread the man greatly," John Carver soberly responded. "We should employ ways and means to safeguard ourselves against him. But how?"

"Why not pen an agreement to be subscribed by all the people?" suggested Stephen Hopkins. "In it we can pledge our allegiance to such officers as we may select and bind ourselves to abide lawfully by their rulings. Once it bears our hands and seals, none can deny at a later date that he has voluntarily submitted himself to the jurisdiction of our laws. It would lay a foundation for our civil government and lend a strong color of authority to all our future acts and deeds."

"Your point is well taken," exclaimed John Carver. "Do you think the London men would subscribe to it?"

"All will do so. John Billington may prove stubborn, but you can count on me to force the issue with him. However, it would be best to dispose of the matter while we're still aboard ship. Once we've landed it might be more difficult to accomplish."

"It shall be done so," John Carver affirmed. "The plan is a most admirable one, and full credit is due you. You've shown yourself to be an able and worthy man. I have no doubt but that you'll stand high in our councils and your advice on matters of state will be heeded second to none."

Stephen Hopkins smiled broadly. "Come then, Mr. Carver. We'll drink a toast to your health."

"Nay, we'll drink one to yours. You've proven by far the better man of the two."

"We'll have no more wrangling," cried Stephen Hopkins with mock severity. "If you must have your way in it, then I must also have mine. We'll drink to each other's health."

Thus, praised be the Lord, the revolt of the London men has been stifled, yet not wholly extinguished, for a few lesser embers still smolder. As for these, they undoubtedly will be kept in check.*

Oh, that Will Butten could have lived to see this blessed day. He died with a foresight of its oncoming, and I for one am secure in the belief that he looked down from his new abode to see its fulfillment. It was no more than a small portion of his just reward. For he was a sacrificial lamb, a martyr to the good of the commonweal.

At the utmost, land is not beyond a day's sail distance. We spent the time to good advantage in cleaning and burnishing our weapons and sharpening our tools for hewing and digging. The people labored cheerfully. Every now and then they would hasten on deck to scan the sea athwart the bow in hope of sighting land prematurely. The oncoming night was our last one at sea, and none spared any regrets over it. The morrow would see us safe in haven. Our long voyage was nearly at its end, and thenceforth we could face our destiny with resolute spirits.

---

* Historical Note: The Mayflower Compact (see *frontispiece*) was signed by 41 of the 49 adult male Pilgrims aboard ship at Cape Cod on November 11, 1620.

Wednesday, November 8, 1620

In the dark of the night long before daybreak I stole a march on our sleeping Company. I was determined to be the first to sight land and stationed myself at the bow to await the dawn with feverish anxiety. It was bitterly cold on deck. A raw wind from the north ate into the marrow and set my teeth chattering. I went below for my cloak and came back to resume my post. The moon and stars were obscured by a clouded sky. I peered intently into the darkness as if to conjure up land before my eyes by the very force of my gaze.

An hour or more went by in solitary observation with nothing to disrupt the stillness or the black walls surrounding me. My impatience mounted with the passage of time. Would dawn never come? Footsteps sounded on the deck to the rear. It was Captain Standish who joined in the vigil with me. The next to appear was John Carver, soon followed by William Brewster and from time to time by others of the people. Each in turn strained his eyes in a futile attempt to pierce the darkness.

After a tedious wait the grey of dawn began sifting in from the east to proclaim the break of day. The dome of heaven lit up, reflecting its light across the sea, and as the veil of night was lifted from the western horizon we redoubled our efforts to sight land.

"What do you see, lad?" inquired Stephen Hopkins at my elbow. "Your eyes are better than mine. Can you see land?"

With hands cupped about my eyes I stared long and earnestly before answering: "Nothing to be seen but the ocean. There's no land in sight."

"Plague take it," he muttered peevishly. "Here I've robbed myself of three to four hours of sleep for no good purpose. I'll warrant Captain Jones has misjudged the distance."

"The light is still dim," I replied. "We'd best wait before we can speak with certainty."

As daylight deepened it failed to reveal more than had originally been disclosed. My own vexation was hardly less than Stephen Hopkins', and after confirming my second finding the people voiced their chagrin in a chorus of disapproval. We had gone to bed last night secure in the thought that land would greet our eyes in the morning. Now it seemed a shadowy promise without hope of fulfillment.

"The day is young," remarked John Carver. "It's not unlikely we'll sight land before nightfall."

"Then Captain Jones should have informed us so," grumbled Stephen Hopkins. "Here he gets us out of bed and keeps us shivering in the frosty air, and to see what? The sea and more sea. I've had my fill of it."

He went below with some of the people to breakfast, their places being taken by others of the Company. I felt no hunger. My blood seethed in anticipation of the great discovery which might ensue any moment. The sun came out astern of us and ascended toward its zenith. We stood rooted at the bow, our eyes ranging far over the sea to the westward. The *Mayflower's* prow cleaved the water and drenched us with showers of cold spray as she sped on to her haven. Several times the cry of "Land!" was raised, but these reports proved groundless. By noonday no trace of land had come to our attention.

The pangs of hunger assailed me. I went below to gulp down a few morsels of food and hastened back on deck, fearful that land might have appeared during my brief absence. The sun had passed its zenith and beat down on the wind-swept sea. White clouds nestling on the western horizon gave a semblance of land and caused false alarms to be sounded. Birds and fowl of varied plumage roved overhead in large numbers. Some of the less timid of these circled so close to the ship that they might have been brought down with muskets.

As the day advanced with no land in the offing, our spirits drooped and many of the people expressed their concern openly.

"I dare say Captain Jones is off the course," Stephen Hopkins averred loudly. "For all we know he may be coasting parallel to the shore to take us northward."

"That could hardly be," said John Carver. "He knows well that he was hired to sail the ship to Hudson's River. I doubt if he would contrive to take us elsewhere."

"I've no faith in sea-captains," declared Stephen Hopkins. "How are we to know if we'll arrive at Hudson's River or anyone else's river, for that matter? Likely as not he'll take us where it's most suitable to his own convenience and let us shift as we're able. We'd best look to ourselves or we'll be the worse for it."

Shortly thereafter Captain Jones made an appearance at the bow.

"How now, Captain Jones?" demanded Stephen Hopkins. "You promised us we'd sight land this day. Here it's nearly nightfall and there isn't even a breath of land. Have you perhaps lost your bearings?"

"I've not lost my bearings," he answered gruffly. "I've sailed the seas too long to be thrown off my course. By my reckoning land is not many leagues away. I'll wager we'll raise it shortly past nightfall or by early daybreak at the latest."

"Another night at sea?" groaned Stephen Hopkins.

"It will be the last," the captain assured him.

"We'll arrive at the mouth of Hudson's River where you were engaged to take us?" inquired John Carver.

"We'll fall in first with Cape Cod. It's like a monstrous hook jutting out from the coast of New England and thence we must sail south by southwest to reach the river. But you need have no fear. The morrow will see us safe in harbor and our journey ended."

"The Lord grant it be so," murmured John Carver.

We again directed our attention to the open sea before

us. It grinned back in malignant mockery of our frustrated desire to reach land. Its countless cohorts, the waves, advanced in serried array against the ship's hull, pounding her keel as if to retard and keep us eternally imprisoned on the deep. At this moment I was strongly impressed with the futility of our puny efforts to transcend distance. The wind and sea were forces for good or evil as their mood suited them. Time alone was our one constant ally. In good season it would aid us to reach our haven.

The sun dipped slowly in the west, submerging itself piecemeal into the sea, and twilight ensued. In the softened afterglow I waited on deck with a few others, gazing westward, ever westward. Toward nightfall I thought I detected a vague, shadowy shore line in the far distance. I uttered a low cry and leaned forward, striving with a last mighty effort to clarify the vision. Then darkness swooped down and all was blurred in my sight.

Thursday, November 9, 1620

I again arose before dawn to await what the new day would bring forth. It was pitch dark on deck; no moon or stars were visible in the sky. I moved forward cautiously and encountered a number of the people already massed at the bow. Some were speaking in eager whispers; others paced to and fro, seeking an outlet for their suppressed agitation. Even in the darkness I sensed the air of expectancy that had aroused them to a fever pitch. Intense hope was aflame in every breast. Land was near at hand. The voyage was almost ended.

The very elements had conspired to kindle within us a feeling of security such as we had never known since our departure from Plymouth. The waves which formerly had been wont to buffet us without mercy were now lapping gently against the hull with a caressing sound. The wind had fallen off with only an occasional gust whistling through the rigging. Having been stripped of sail, the ship lay becalmed as she rose and fell easily in the swell of the sea. It was as though we were resting safely in harbor, free from the dangers which had harried us unceasingly these past two months and more.

As daybreak neared, the tension was bloated to the bursting point. All speech and movement were hushed in a deathlike silence. The people were hunched forward like so many frozen images, intent on conserving their vigor for the welcome sight of land and the glad outcry to follow in the wake of discovery. The heavy, muffled respirations of those about me resounded in my ears. My own breath came in short, quick gasps, and I felt the blood coursing through my veins like the current from a seething whirlpool.

The first shafts of light filtered through with maddening deliberation. Slowly a view of the western horizon was unfolded and stood partly revealed in the murky haze. For the second successive morning I cupped my hands about my eyes and gazed straight before me. There to the westward was a long, thin line reaching northward and southward. It might have been a breaker, and I paused for a few precious seconds to reassure myself. Then as the gloom was somewhat dispelled, it appeared as clear and distinct a stretch of shore as could be expected in the dubious light.

"Land ahead," I cried out in exultation.

Instantly the stillness of morning was ruptured by the rattle of musketry and a volley of shouts.

"Land, land, land!"

It rose and swelled into a mighty volume, reverberating over the sea in a deafening outburst and soaring upward to heaven itself. There it was, the Land of Canaan, the Promised Land, the Land of Milk and Honey. The people could not contain themselves for joy. They laughed and cried, danced and sang, and gave praise to the Lord for having delivered them from the perils of the sea and brought them safely to their journey's end. It was a moment of abandonment to sheer rejoicing mingled with fervent thanksgiving, a recompense for the many sore trials and desperate ordeals we had undergone.

The first flush of mad acclaim having subsided, our attention was again drawn to the land before us. On closer approach we observed it extended north and south beyond the uttermost limits of our vision, a pleasant, verdant country, heavily wooded with virginal forests as yet untouched by the inroads of man. Trees and foliage grew down to the water's edge and thence ran inland far back from the sea. For the main part the branches were bare, yet some were still covered with leaves in autumnal tresses of yellow, brown and gold, and these seemed to beckon to us in friendly welcome. Truly, wanderers that we were upon the face of the earth, we felt ourselves home at last and gave thanks to the Lord that this, our country to be, seemed so fertile and promising a land for habitation.

The people feasted their eyes as if they would never be satiated and plied Captain Jones with an uninterrupted flow of questions. He, poor man, was beset on all sides at one and the same time, not knowing where to turn or whom to answer first. The substance of his replies was to the effect that we were indeed at Cape Cod and by coasting along the shore a few leagues to the northwest we

could round the northern extremity of the cape and arrive
at a good harbor in a great bay called Cape Cod Bay. He
further related it had been so named because of the
abundance of cod fish in its waters; also it was reputed to
be a favorite nesting haunt for innumerable birds and
fowl, and the nearby woods abounded in game of all sorts.

His narration exceeded our fondest hopes and whetted
our desire to land forthwith fully as much as our yearning
to tread firm earth again. We had been overly long at sea
and were weary of being wind-and-wave tossed. Here was
a land of plenty with a threefold source of meat for our
victuals. To judge from the bounteous plant life, the soil
must be fertile for the growing of crops. What reason
was there to seek a better place for our habitation? Thus
ran the discourse, and many of the people were eager to
round the cape and put into harbor without delay.

In response to the clamor, our chief men consulted
earnestly among themselves and with Captain Jones. I
could not follow the discussion in its entirety. In favor
of landing at once, it was observed that the country about
Cape Cod seemed a hopeful place and suitable in many
ways for our settlement; also, wintry weather would assail
us before long and it was doubtful if much time could be
spent in beating about near Hudson's River in search of
a habitation. On the other hand, the original intention
had been to settle in the region of Hudson's River. It was
feared that our land grant restricted us to the northern
parts of Virginia and would be void at Cape Cod or any

other part of New England. This was a sobering thought which called for grave deliberation.

The upshot was that we were to stand by our first resolve and go to the mouth of Hudson's River. Without delay the sail was hoisted and trimmed to the breeze, the ship was tacked to a southerly course and we started off with a fair wind. The people were clustered at the starboard bow, sorrowful and dejected at the thought of departing from the pleasant country. From what we had seen and heard of Cape Cod we were loath to leave it, yet no voices were raised in protest.

We sailed along the shore of Cape Cod, finding it an ever constant source of admiration. Coves and snug little bays indented the coast, small ponds and rivers wound from the interior to empty into the sea, and everywhere endless forests of sweet woods flourished. Some of the trees we distinguished as oak, maple, birch and pine; others seemed to bear no resemblance to our English trees. The country was fairly level, being barren of mountains, hills and valleys. We observed no inhabitants, savage or otherwise, and no signs of habitation. For all we could see, it was a virgin land as yet untrodden and unconquered.

By midday we had covered some eight to ten leagues, and Captain Jones announced that before long we would round the southeastern extremity of Cape Cod and thence sail southwest to Hudson's River. At this point the lookout shouted a warning of breakers ahead. Off the mainland to the south, the sea was dotted with numerous small islands, leaving a scant channel for clearance. Between the mainland and the islands, the water seethed and churned in turmoil like a veritable whirlpool. The roar of breakers dinned in our ears with increasing volume as we drew near.

Robert Coppin, the pilot, stationed himself at the bow, fathom line in hand to plumb the depths, and foot by foot we sounded our way forward. The endeavor was fraught with peril of no uncertain degree, sending our hearts to our mouths. Time and again it was feared the *Mayflower* would be grounded on the shoals or her keel would strike on the rocks submerged in the water. Slowly she crept onward at a snail's pace, barely escaping one danger after another by the scantest of hairbreadths. The pilot's voice rang out shrilly above the tumult of the breakers as he told off the depth and directed our course.

We had covered almost half of the difficult passage when a new hazard ensued. The wind fell off, leaving the ship becalmed in the midst of the swirling water and buffeted about at the mercy of the furious eddies and currents. Instantly the seamen let fall three anchors to hold her in place; whichever way she tugged, the lines held her safe from the teeth of the shoals. For the time we were secure, but our position was far from being an enviable one. There we were in a raging vortex, clinging to dear life by the grace of God and three anchors.

We were ensnared in this pitfall for fully three hours

without a breath of wind; then it began to blow West South West. Again our chief men consulted with Captain Jones as to our best expedient. The wind being opposite, we could make no sail to the southwest and it was concluded to abandon our design to settle near Hudson's River and instead to bear up for Cape Cod. These tidings were received with an outburst of cheers from the people. Cape Cod had taken all our hearts by storm and we were overjoyed at the thought of returning thereto for our habitation.

The ship was tacked about and we cautiously retraced our way out of the turbulent waters. It was almost nightfall before this was accomplished, but with the Lord's aid it was done in safety. Out in the clear, full sail was unfurled and we thankfully watched the treacherous shoals waxing dim in our wake as we sped northward. We were homeward bound. A benignant moon smiled down on us and lit up our environs in a glow of serenity. And standing hand-in-hand at the bow, Elizabeth and I gazed hopefully before us as the *Mayflower* bore us nearer and nearer to haven.